READMISSION PREVENTION

JOSH D. LUKE

READMISSION PREVENTION

SOLUTIONS ACROSS THE PROVIDER CONTINUUM

ACHE Management Series

Library of Congress Cataloging-in-Publication Data

Luke, Josh D., author.
  Readmission prevention : solutions across the provider continuum / Josh D. Luke.
    p. ; cm. — (ACHE management series)
  Includes bibliographical references.
  ISBN 978-1-56793-710-7 (alk. paper)
  I. Title. II. Series: Management series (Ann Arbor, Mich.)
  [DNLM: 1. Patient Readmission—United States. 2. Hospitals—standards—United States. 3. Quality Improvement—United States. WX 158]
  HG9389.H6
  368.38'27—dc23
                          2014044636

The paper used in this publication meets the minimum requirements of American National Standard for Information Sciences—Permanence of Paper for Printed Library Materials, ANSI Z39.48-1984. ∞™

Acquisitions editor: Tulie O'Connor; Project editor: Andrew Baumann; Cover designer: David Orr; Layout: PerfecType

Found an error or a typo? We want to know! Please e-mail it to hapbooks@ache.org and put "Book Error" in the subject line.

For photocopying and copyright information, please contact Copyright Clearance Center at www.copyright.com or (978) 750-8400.

Health Administration Press
A division of the Foundation of the American
    College of Healthcare Executives
One North Franklin Street, Suite 1700
Chicago, IL 60606-3529
(312) 424-2800

Contents

Part I: Defining Readmissions and Their Impact on the Healthcare Delivery System

   *Hospital Readmission: A Practical Definition •
   Historical Background of the Readmission Problem •
   What Causes Hospital Readmissions? • All-Cause
   Readmissions • The Readmission Problem • Readmission
   Trends 2010 to 2013 • Tactical Approaches to the
   Readmission Problem*

   *The "Putting Heads in Beds" Mind-Set • The Problem
   of Observation Days • Collecting Readmission Data •
   No Cookie-Cutter Answers*

   Perspective: The Impact of ICD-9-CM and ICD-10
   on Readmission Measurement Under the ACA
   by James S. Kennedy, MD

Part II: The Three Phases of Preparation to Prevent Readmissions

Part III: Transitional Care Programs and Models

Part IV: Readmission Prevention Models by Level of Care

Teach-Back Methods • Pursue Contract Alignment • Conduct Genetic Testing • Narrow the Home Health Network and Coordinate Home Health Services • Adopt INTERACT Tools • Implement Direct-from-ED and Observation Unit Transfers • Summary

Perspective: Using Post-Acute Care Venues to Reduce Readmissions *by Cherilyn G. Murer, JD*

Make Sure POLST Forms Are Available for All Patients • Conduct or Gain Access to Patient Risk Assessments • Participate in Post-Acute Care Networks and Community Collaboratives • Make Sure You Are Part of the Hospital's Narrow Network • Identify Local Transitional Care Programs • Provide Ambulatory Case Management Services • Provide Remote Monitoring Services • Collect Facility-Specific Data • Connect via a Health Information Exchange • Have a Consistent Marketing Plan • Promote Self-Management, Patient Health Literacy, and Use of Teach-Back Methods • Pursue Contract Alignment • Conduct Genetic Testing • Adopt INTERACT Tools • Triage the Patient When an Acute Care Episode Occurs • Refer All Patients to Home Care or Private-Duty Nursing on Discharge • Implement Transfers Directly from the ED to Home with Home Health Services • Summary

Perspective: Rehabilitation Is Vital in Readmission Prevention *by Sarah Thomas*

Make Sure POLST Forms Are Available for All Patients • Conduct or Gain Access to Patient Risk Assessments • Participate in Post-Acute Care Networks and Community

Collaboratives • Make Sure You Are Part of the Hospital's Narrow Network • Identify Local Transitional Care Programs • Provide Ambulatory Case Management Services • Provide Remote Monitoring Services • Collect Facility-Specific Data • Connect via a Health Information Exchange • Have a Consistent Marketing Plan • Triage the Patient When an Acute Care Episode Occurs • Implement Transfers Directly from the ED to Home with Hospice or Palliative Care • Summary

Perspective: The Pharmacist's Role in Readmission Prevention: Medication Therapy Management *by Kerjun Chang, PharmD, and Sheetal Amin, PharmD*

Perspective: The Role of Hospice and Palliative Care in Readmissions *by Alen Voskanian, MD*

Make Sure POLST Forms Are Available for All Patients • Conduct or Gain Access to Patient Risk Assessments • Participate in Post-Acute Care Networks and Community Collaboratives • Make Sure You Are Part of the Hospital's Narrow Network • Identify Local Transitional Care Programs • Provide Ambulatory Case Management Services • Provide Remote Monitoring Services • Collect Facility-Specific Data • Connect via a Health Information Exchange • Have a Consistent Marketing Plan • Promote Self-Management, Patient Health Literacy, and Use of Teach-Back Methods • Pursue Contract Alignment • Conduct Genetic Testing • Narrow the Home Health Network and Coordinate Home Health Services • Adopt INTERACT Tools • Invest in Predictive Software • Implement Direct-from-ED and Observation Unit Transfers • Summary

Perspective: Helping Patients and Their Caregivers Find Hope in Realistic Healthcare Goals *by Nicholas Jauregui, MD*

Make Sure POLST Forms Are Available for All Patients • Conduct or Gain Access to Patient Risk Assessments • Participate in Post-Acute Care Networks and Community Collaboratives • Make Sure You Are Part of the Hospital's Narrow Network • Identify Local Transitional Care Programs • Provide Ambulatory Case Management Services • Provide Remote Monitoring Services • Collect Agency-Specific Data • Connect via a Health Information Exchange • Have a Consistent Marketing Plan • Promote Self-Management, Patient Health Literacy, and Use of Teach-Back Methods • Pursue Contract Alignment • Triage the Patient When an Acute Care Episode Occurs • Refer All Patients to Home Care or Private-Duty Nursing on Discharge from Home Health • Implement Transfers Directly from the ED to Home with Home Care or Private-Duty Nurse Support • Equip Family Members and Friends to Serve as Caretakers • Summary

Perspective: Preventing Readmissions Through Home Visits *by Jay Licuanan, MD*

Perspective: Reducing Psychiatric Readmissions from the Emergency Department *by Leslie S. Zun, MD*

Part V: Epilogue

Foreword

The task of hospital readmission prevention is shrouded in myths. One myth states that readmission is a passing fad and, as such, warrants only short-term quick fixes. A second myth maintains that hospital readmissions largely result from the behavior of non-compliant patients. A third myth upholds the position that reducing readmissions is a problem for the hospital to solve alone. And finally, a fourth myth tries to convince us that the primary reason for focusing on readmission prevention is simply to avoid penalties.

Thus, it is with great anticipation that I introduce an important contribution to the field, *Readmission Prevention: Solutions Across the Provider Continuum.* Consider this your trusted myth-busting handbook. Some of the most respected thought leaders in the field offer broad-based strategies for how clinicians and organizations can excel in an era of value-based payment and population care. This action-oriented guide emanates not from the ivory tower but rather from the practical lessons that can only be gleaned from the front lines.

Trial and error have served only to reinforce the humbling observation that there are no quick fixes in readmission prevention. Thus, what impresses me most about this book is that it embraces a comprehensive and multifaceted approach. Previously, this wealth of information could not be found in any one place.

After immersing yourself in the upcoming chapters, you undoubtedly will gain the knowledge, skills, and tools you need to execute a successful readmission prevention program. Read on!

Eric A. Coleman, MD, MPH
Director, Care Transitions Program

Preface

Are readmission penalties enough to spur hospitals to action? The answer, unfortunately, is no. Readmission penalties alone are not enough to get hospitals to focus on value-based reimbursement and create coordinated care models. However, considering that the Affordable Care Act (ACA) of 2010 includes six initiatives specific to coordinating care between providers—two incentives (accountable care organizations and bundled-payment initiatives) and four penalties (readmission penalties, recovery audits, the Medicare Spending per Beneficiary measure, and other value-based purchasing opportunities)—the combined impact of these six initiatives is enough to encourage hospitals and health systems to implement value-based coordinated care models. However, it's going to take time.

After I earned a master's degree in public relations in 1996, I found my dream job in sports marketing. I had grown up a huge sports fan, a junkie if you will, playing three sports in high school and scrumming it up daily in the front yard (any shape or size ball would do) with my two older brothers, Scott and Matt. Although my two older brothers are blessed with greater athletic ability, I share their love for just about every sport.

In 1998, just a few days after slugger Mark McGwire broke the single-season home-run record of 61, through hard work and a stroke of good luck the global public relations firm I was working for was hired to handle the new home-run king's personal marketing and public relations. I was appointed account lead and, a few weeks later, found myself on a private jet with McGwire and some of his closest friends. I escorted him to interviews with *Time* magazine (which was considering him as a "Man of the Year" candidate), the *Today Show*, *The Late Show with David Letterman*, and *The Rosie O'Donnell Show*.

Though my experiences in sports marketing were exciting, it was the events of the next few years that would change my life. By the summer of 2001, I was feeling unfulfilled in my career. At the same time, my beloved grandmother's congestive heart failure was proving too much for her to handle. Belva Mae Riddle, who had a beautiful mind and was one of the most caring and strongest-willed people you could ever meet, began a cycle of bouncing back and forth between the hospital, a nursing home, and her home that would last several years.

I was living several hundred miles away, completing my graduate studies, and my frequent calls home to California to check on my grandmother often led to frustration. I was perplexed at how caretakers at the hospital and nursing home communicated so little with each other when my grandmother transferred from one facility to the other. I was even more shocked to find that when she would return home, the home-based caretakers seemed to have few instructions from the hospital or nursing home. My frustration was growing.

I was teaching a night course at a local university, and one evening a student approached me after class to ask if I would be interested in applying for the position of director of marketing and admissions for a local skilled-nursing facility. Initially, it seemed like too huge a leap in my career path, but through much prayer and discussion with my wife, I decided to apply. Life Care Centers of America is a reputable organization with facilities throughout the country, and it has an administrator-in-training (AIT) program designed to teach young professionals to be future healthcare leaders and operators.

I still was not convinced the nursing home industry was the change I had been waiting for, but the defining moment in my life and career took place as I entered the front doors of Life Care Center of Reno, Nevada. In the entry sat an elderly woman who appeared to be unaware of her surroundings; she was slouched over and slipping from her wheelchair. Not knowing if she needed assistance or not, I stood in my tracks and pondered my next move. Should I help her? Is this normal for her? Is she in pain? I did not know the answers to these questions, but I did know this situation would shape and define who I would become as a healthcare leader.

God undoubtedly put this elderly woman in the entry that day to challenge me to stop and consider the task ahead. And though I did not know if she was in pain or needed help, that moment drove my decision to change my career. I approached her, bent down to her eye level, and with a smile asked if I could help her with anything. She said she was doing fine, thanked me for asking, and smiled as I walked away. This was my first lesson as a healthcare administrator: The patient's needs and care are always your top priority—regardless of how busy you are that day. Wearing your servant's heart on your sleeve at all times is nonnegotiable.

That moment with the elderly woman in the entry and later walking into the nursing home for my first day of work were two of the most humbling experiences of my life. They shaped me as a leader and, most important, gave me personal confirmation of my servant's heart. Not only would I be serving as director of marketing and admissions for Life Care Center, but I had also been accepted into the AIT program. And just like that, I made a career change—a change that was instigated by my grandmother, of all people.

When I was a young administrator, I often told the story of how my grandmother's struggles led me to a new career path. Little did I know that about ten years later, when I was traveling the country to speak about the topics of readmissions, care coordination, and population health management, I would once again share her negative hospital readmission experiences as a perfect example of why our healthcare system needed to be transformed. Fifteen years to the month after that private jet trip to New York with Mark McGwire, I was asked to be the executive chair of an annual event in Orlando—the World Congress Leadership Summit on Readmission Prevention. That role was a far cry from taking sports celebrities on media tours, but it was a position I was honored to serve in.

I have a great passion for the readmission issue, and I am sure you will see many examples of that passion throughout this book. Readmission penalties are one of at least six initiatives in the ACA designed to incentivize coordinated care. This book will focus specifically on proven tactics to prevent unnecessary hospital read-missions. Naturally, improved coordinated care efforts and models are the end result of effective readmission prevention strategies. However, there is already a significant body of literature on care coordination models. Thus, this book attempts to look specifically at ways to prevent unnecessary hospital readmissions by collaborating with post-acute care providers at all levels to make sure patients are hospitalized only when their needs cannot be met at a lower level of care.

My experiences as CEO of several acute care and acute rehabilitation hospitals, vice president of a health system (overseeing hospice and home health), and administrator of multiple skilled-nursing and assisted-living facilities give me a thorough foundation for writing this book. In addition to providing my own viewpoints, I have drawn on the expertise and knowledge of several trusted friends and colleagues from around the country to provide best practices and proven tactics to prevent unnecessary hospital readmissions. My goal is to show you how to best address the readmission issue by developing an effective and strategic population management program designed specifically for your community and hospital.

Acknowledgments

My preparation for becoming a published author started in high school when one of my most influential teachers, the late Shaun Hulbert, kept digging at my core until he found the means to turn my passion for life into a passion for literature and writing. Connie Grosse, another of my former high school teachers, continues to carry that torch of keeping me motivated even today.

When I was in college, my father fought for me to have the opportunity to get an education even though having four kids in college at the same time was a tremendous financial burden. It was my mother's voice, however, that I needed to hear every day on the other end of the phone line to keep me going and feeling loved.

In the early years of our marriage, my dear wife Martine supported my goal of earning a PhD even though it meant her being home alone a few nights a week (receiving a Labrador puppy as a Christmas gift solved that problem). More important, I am grateful that she has supported me unconditionally as my innovative ideas and vision came to fruition, no matter how crazy they sounded at times. I could not have completed this project without the love and support of my best friend and wife of more than 15 years.

I am thankful to the people at Life Care Centers of America who gave me my first job in healthcare as a nursing home marketer and administrator in training. I owe the most respect and gratitude to R. Michael Hartman, a seasoned health system vice president who had the confidence in me to give me my first hospital CEO job. I am also grateful to healthcare executives Dr. Mark Bell, Dan Brothman, Craig Leach, Arnie Schaffer, and Jim Young for having the confidence in me to appoint me to C-suite positions in their organizations as well.

I would like to thank the up-and-coming healthcare executives who served as volunteers when I founded the National Readmission Prevention Collaborative—most specifically Courtney Downey, Beth Garcia, Corri Holm, Elaine Lombardi, Martine Luke, Wendy

Cohn Luke, Katie Mannino, Ebinehita Omofoma, and Lodel Yerro. I would also like to thank Jim Riemenschneider of COMS Interactive for inspiring me to move forward with my vision of forming the collaborative and its website. Were it not for the innovative tools and solutions COMS Interactive created to improve the coordinated care model, my message would be void of answers and direction for those who seek to improve the continuum of care.

I would like to thank the industry experts who submitted Perspectives essays for this book as well as those who spent their valuable time reviewing and editing the book, including Courtney Downey, Mike Hartman, and Shawn Noetzli. I would also like to thank Eric Coleman, whom I consider to be the most respected and authoritative figure in the readmissions prevention space, for generously agreeing to write the foreword. Thanks, too, to the American College of Healthcare Executives and Health Administration Press for accepting this book for publication and to all the staff there who supported me in making it happen.

Finally, I dedicate this book to my grandparents and my mother, all of whom have been challenged by Alzheimer's disease. I am committed to redefining our healthcare delivery system to a patient-centered model so that future generations will receive a level of care that is more comprehensive than the fragmented model my grandparents and mother struggled through. I hope my contribution to the evolution of this patient-centered model will someday be my legacy. This book is a small step in that direction.

Introduction

The goal of this book is simple: to provide a user-friendly guide for healthcare operators to implement tactics to prevent unnecessary hospital readmissions. I hope these tactics prove useful in your facility or agency—as well as within your community.

By reading this book and implementing a few of the readmission prevention tactics described, acute care hospital operators should see a significant decline in their hospital's readmission rate and the readmission penalty administered annually by the Centers for Medicare & Medicaid Services. Furthermore, operators of post-acute care facilities or agencies can implement the tactics in this book to help a referring hospital reduce its unnecessary readmission rate and position itself as the provider of choice in the community. Under the new provisions of the Affordable Care Act, it is more important than ever for post-acute care providers to take the steps needed to be a provider of choice as hospitals, health systems, and managed care organizations narrow their networks aggressively to work with a select few preferred providers.

In the past few years I have had the privilege of meeting and exchanging ideas and experiences with some of the greatest minds in the readmission world and the developers of fantastic transition programs. These thought leaders and innovators include Eric Coleman, MD, MPH, creator of the Care Transitions Intervention; Kathryn Bowles, MSN, PhD, who pioneered what I believe to be the most comprehensive and accurate electronic risk assessment tool available; and Stephen Jencks, MD, whom I refer to as the godfather and inventor of the readmission issue. I have great respect for the physicians and scientists who pioneered these care transition models and encourage you to research their work further. Yet, while their programs are detailed and effective and all have improved the value-based care model, many hospitals, health systems, and communities do not have the resources necessary to implement comprehensive transitional care programs. Thus, I wanted to take a different approach with this book.

I served seven years as CEO for a safety-net hospital, where we cared for the neediest of the needy, including the homeless and adult psychiatric patients. This experience shaped me as a healthcare administrator and inspired me to write this book. In this world, providers fight for those without a voice, those whose care needs are often forgotten because they are unable to pay for the services they receive. My goal is to provide a comprehensive list of individual readmission prevention tactics in hopes that one or two of them might work in your healthcare facility, even if you have no budget for such programs. I envision that readers will keep a marker handy at all times to highlight tactics that might prove useful in preventing unnecessary hospital readmissions in their particular hospital or community and then create a list of those that stood out as compatible with their needs.

The book includes a chapter written specifically for hospital operators. In addition, post-acute care administrators and operators will find specific chapters for each level of post-acute care, including skilled nursing and home health. Having served as an executive or administrator in several of these areas of care, I have aimed to speak to the specific business goals and objectives of each, to provide new and innovative strategies to prevent unnecessary hospital readmissions, and to help operators position their facility or agency as the provider of choice in the community.

Throughout this book you will find short Perspectives sections that were written by experts in the healthcare field to provide additional viewpoints on critical issues in care transitions. Although I have a comprehensive understanding of the care continuum as a whole, I thought inviting the opinions of experts in each specialty area might provide additional insights on how avoidable readmissions can be managed at different levels of post-acute care.

My intent has been to write a book that is user-friendly, conversational, and tactical, not one that is resource oriented and overladen with data and statistics. Of course, I cannot provide an effective tool kit to prevent unnecessary hospital readmissions without first identifying the problem, how it originated, and the specifics of the readmission penalty, and that will be covered in Chapter 1.

Abbreviations

3MHIS	3M Health Information Systems
ACA	Affordable Care Act
ACM	ambulatory case manager
ACO	accountable care organization
AIT	administrator in training
AMI	acute myocardial infarction
APR-DRG	all-payer-refined diagnosis-related group
BCC	bridge care coordinator
BOOST	Better Outcomes for Older Adults through Safe Transitions
CHF	congestive heart failure
CMS	Centers for Medicare & Medicaid Services
COPD	chronic obstructive pulmonary disease
CPT	Current Procedural Terminology
CTI	Care Transitions Interventions
DRG	diagnosis-related group
ED	emergency department
FY	fiscal year
GRACE	Geriatric Resources for Assessment and Care of Elders
HCC	Hierarchical Condition Category
HIE	health information exchange
HIPAA	Health Insurance Portability and Accountability Act
HRRP	Hospital Readmission Reduction Program
ICD-9-CM	International Classification of Diseases, Ninth Revision, Clinical Modification
ICD-10-CM	International Classification of Diseases, Tenth Revision, Clinical Modification
INTERACT	Interventions to Reduce Acute Care Transfers
IPPS	Inpatient Prospective Payment System
IRF	inpatient rehabilitation facility

JOC	joint operating committee
LANE	Local Area Network for Excellence
LTAC	long-term acute care
MedPAC	Medicare Payment Advisory Commission
MSPB	Medicare Spending per Beneficiary
MTM	medication therapy management
NTOCC	National Transitions of Care Coalition
O/E ratio	observed-to-expected ratio
PACT	Post-Acute Care Transitions
PEPPER	Program for Evaluating Payment Patterns Electronic Report
POLST	Physician Orders for Life-Sustaining Treatment
PPR	potentially preventable readmission
RAC	Recovery Audit Contractor
REACH	Reconciliation, Education, Access, Counseling, Healthy Patient at Home
RED	Re-Engineered Discharge
SBAR	situation, background, assessment, and recommendation
SHM	Society of Hospital Medicine
SNF	skilled-nursing facility
SOI	severity of illness
STAAR	State Action on Avoidable Rehospitalization
SWOT	strengths, weaknesses, opportunities, threats
TCM	Transitional Care Model
TRAC	Tenet Readmission Advisory Committee
UHC	University HealthSystem Consortium

Part I

DEFINING READMISSIONS AND THEIR IMPACT ON THE HEALTHCARE DELIVERY SYSTEM

CHAPTER 1

The Affordable Care Act and the Readmission Problem

This chapter provides a historical perspective on how readmissions were identified as a concern and how the issue has evolved since the Hospital Readmission Reduction Program (HRRP) was introduced in October 2012 (see Exhibit 1.1 for a timeline of the program's implementation). The chapter is more data driven than the rest of the book because a quantitative perspective is necessary to understand the readmission problem.

HOSPITAL READMISSION: A PRACTICAL DEFINITION

As it pertains to the penalty program, the Affordable Care Act (ACA 2010, §3025) defines a readmission as a person being admitted to the same or a different acute care hospital within 30 days of discharge from the initial hospital stay. The initial hospital stay is referred to as the *index stay*. The readmission penalty applies to all Medicare fee-for-service beneficiaries except those enrolled in a Medicare Advantage program, those enrolled in Part A or Part B only, and those who age in after January.

Exhibit 1.1 Implementation Timeline for the Hospital Readmission Reduction Program (HRRP)

Data Period	Timeline
FY 2013	July 2008 to June 2011
HRRP preview reports posted to QNet (includes AMI, CHF, and pneumonia)	June 2012
HRRP penalty calculations published	August 2012
Penalties up to 1% (up to 1% of all base DRG payments)	Beginning October 1, 2012
FY 2014	July 2009 to June 2012
HRRP preview reports posted to QNet (includes AMI, CHF, and pneumonia)	June 2013
HRRP penalty calculations published	August 2013
Penalties up to 2% (up to 2% of all base DRG payments)	Beginning October 1, 2013
FY 2015	July 2010 to June 2013
HRRP preview reports posted to QNet (includes AMI, CHF, pneumonia, COPD, and total knee and hip surgery)	June 2014
HRRP penalty calculations published	August 2014
Penalties up to 3% (up to 3% of all base DRG payments)	Beginning October 1, 2014

Source: Adapted from ACA (2010), §3025.

Notes: FY = fiscal year; DRG = diagnosis-related group; AMI = acute myocardial infarction; CHF = congestive heart failure; COPD = chronic obstructive pulmonary disease.

In short, the entire readmission penalty program is simply the stroke of a key in the Medicare Inpatient Prospective Payment System (IPPS) database. At the end of the year, the IPPS database spits out a report that lists all patients who were discharged from an acute care hospital and subsequently admitted to the same or another acute care hospital within 30 days. Regardless of the reason the patient is readmitted to the hospital, the readmission counts against the hospital that originally discharged the patient during the index stay. The patient's primary discharge diagnosis during the index stay determines the disease-specific classification of the penalty.

For example, suppose Jane, a Medicare fee-for-service patient, is admitted to her hometown hospital with pneumonia. After four days she is discharged to a skilled-nursing facility for two weeks and then is discharged home. All of the caretakers across the continuum of care met and exceeded the care plan goals, and Jane returned home safely. One week later she drives three hours to attend her grandson's graduation from college. On the way, she is in a car accident and is admitted to the local hospital. Although the second stay is not related to the initial diagnosis of pneumonia, it counts as a readmission against her hometown hospital, which cared for her during the index stay.

HISTORICAL BACKGROUND OF THE READMISSION PROBLEM

The Centers for Medicare & Medicaid Services (CMS), which has been studying the problem of unnecessary hospital readmissions for years, believes the continued increase in readmission rates signifies a decline in the quality of care being provided at hospitals nationwide (Khan 2013). Of about 31 million Medicare beneficiaries, each year approximately 4 percent, or 1.2 million patients, are readmitted to the hospital within 30 days (CMS 2014). Such readmissions cost the Medicare program approximately $17.5 billion in inpatient spending in 2010 (ACA 2010, §3025). Furthermore, the CMS spends an estimated $11,200 per readmission, and the current all-cause readmission rate is 21.2 percent (Rizzo 2013).

The ACA introduced penalties for acute care hospitals with excessive readmissions under Medicare's IPPS (ACA 2010, §3025). In 2007, the Medicare Payment Advisory Commission (MedPAC) identified seven conditions and procedures that accounted for almost 30 percent of preventable readmissions, and CMS worked in conjunction with the National Quality Forum to identify three of these disease categories—acute myocardial infarction, congestive heart failure, and pneumonia—that would be included in the initial readmission penalty for fiscal year (FY) 2013 (ACA 2010, §3025; CMA 2014). For FY 2015, CMS expanded the readmission penalty to include two more disease-specific categories, chronic obstructive pulmonary disease (COPD) and knee and hip surgeries.

Although the initial ACA legislation had exclusions for planned readmissions for a number of diagnosis codes, planned surgeries, or transfers to another hospital, the hospital community perceived the list of exclusions to be very small (ACA 2010, §3025). The CMS expanded the list of exclusions for FY 2015 when it added COPD and total knee and hip replacement (*Federal Register* 2013). Studying and understanding these exclusions can be a complicated process, and most hospitals and health systems do not have the resources to invest in such studies. To date, the financial penalties for unnecessary hospital readmissions have not been significant enough in most cases to justify such research.

CMS will reduce a hospital's diagnosis-related group (DRG) payments when the hospital's readmission ratio is exceeded, with respect to payment for discharges from the hospital. The financial penalty amounted to a reduction to 0.99 in FY 2013, 0.98 in FY 2014, and 0.97 in FY 2015 (CMA 2014). As of the time of writing, CMS has not indicated that it will further reduce hospitals' DRG payments beyond the 0.97 reduction. However, it is widely speculated that CMS will either continue to reduce hospitals' DRG payments on the basis of excessive readmissions or expand the penalty to additional disease-specific categories after FY 2015. See Exhibit 1.2 for statistics on the financial impact of hospital readmissions.

Because the hospital community has not made significant strides or efforts to address the readmission problem, CMS will likely continue to seek ways to penalize hospitals for admitting patients who could be cared for at lower levels of care, even beyond the six programs in the ACA that incentivize hospitals and health systems to coordinate care.

WHAT CAUSES HOSPITAL READMISSIONS?

According to a study by the Dartmouth Institute, patients are readmitted to the hospital for five primary reasons (Khan 2013):

1. Patients may not fully understand what is wrong with them.
2. Patients may be confused over which medications to take and when to take them.
3. Hospitals do not provide the patient or doctors with important information or test results.
4. Patients do not schedule a follow-up appointment with their doctor.
5. Family members lack the proper knowledge to provide adequate care.

Research indicates that readmissions for these primary reasons are likely avoidable across facilities nationwide. Breakdowns in communication, lack of formal structure for discharge planning, and a lack of emphasis on coordinating care between levels of care have led to readmission rates that are costly because they are unnecessary and preventable (Abrams and Levy 2013).

Exhibit 1.2. Financial Impact of Hospital Readmissions

	Congestive Heart Failure	Acute Myocardial Infarction	Pneumonia	Chronic Obstructive Pulmonary Disease	Joint Replacement
Cost per readmission	$13,000	$13,200	$13,000	$8,400	$12,300
Readmission rate	25.1%	17.1%	15.3%	7.1%	8.2%
Cost of initial admission	$11,000	$20,800	$9,600	$7,100	$10,200
Percentage of cost of initial admission	118%	64%	135%	118%	121%

Sources: Adapted from Elixhauser, Au, and Podulka (2011) and Qasim and Andrews (2012).

In addition to a reimbursement model that has incentivized physicians, hospitals, and all levels of post-acute care to admit patients and use services, socioeconomic factors are often a greater driver of readmissions to the hospital than clinical issues are. In particular, for senior citizens who may live alone, lack of food in the refrigerator, insufficient financial resources to fill prescriptions, inadequate understanding of the medication regimen, or unavailability of transportation to the pharmacy, grocery store, or doctor's appointment often lead to unnecessary hospital readmissions. More important, patient literacy and self-management are the most critical factors in preventing unnecessary hospital admissions. This book will provide a series of tactics to address each of those critical factors, whether clinically or socially based.

ALL-CAUSE READMISSIONS

Many facilities nationwide have implemented disease-specific readmission prevention programs, and many of these programs have been successful in preventing unnecessary hospital readmissions. That said, this book focuses almost exclusively on tactics that providers at all levels of care can implement to prevent all-cause readmissions.

A number of best-practice case studies are provided at the end of this book to showcase many of these all-cause tactics and programs. A few of the case studies highlight disease-specific programs for readers interested in a more linear approach to the problem.

One of the reasons this book focuses on all-cause readmissions is that few health systems and hospitals have the resources to implement multiple disease-specific programs. Many hospitals have attempted to implement multiple programs only to find that the different approaches and tactics proved confusing to many of the caretakers, and thus none of the individual programs was sustainable.

As noted, starting in FY 2015 hospitals are being penalized for readmissions in five disease-specific categories. Hospitals are also now evaluated on their all-cause readmission rate for Medicare fee-for-service patients. Although hospitals' all-cause readmission rates were not initially included in the penalty program, all-cause readmissions are included in the inpatient quality-reporting program. Hospitals are not financially penalized for each disease-specific readmission but rather for an accumulation of readmissions in each of the five disease-specific categories. Therefore, by taking a facility-wide and organization-wide approach to the problem, hospitals and health systems should be able to implement effective comprehensive readmission prevention programs.

THE READMISSION PROBLEM

To simplify readmissions, the Medicare fee-for-service model incentivized facilities to admit patients. Medicare fee-for-service also incentivized physicians to admit patients to the hospital, skilled-nursing facilities, long-term acute care hospitals, acute rehabilitation hospitals, and home health agencies by reimbursing them each time they admitted a patient to one of these levels of care. Often, physicians could be reimbursed every day while caring for such patients. Likewise, hospitals were incentivized to admit patients to all levels of care. Quite simply, no system of checks and balances was in place under the fee-for-service model. I call this era the "fee-for-service free-for-all."

Although this era was a lucrative time for many hospitals, facilities, physicians, and home health agencies, it ultimately put the federal government in a compromising position as funds for healthcare ran dry. The ACA, though far from perfect, was a historic attempt to change the way care is delivered in the United States. Clearly, the desired model is a coordinated care model that leaves the fee-for-service free-for-all in the past. The model is designed to reimburse physicians and providers for care based on value and quality rather than for episodic care whenever a patient needs to be hospitalized.

In 2003, such a model would have incentivized caretakers at all levels to collaborate to improve outcomes instead of viewing and treating all patients, my grandmother included, as commodities.

READMISSION TRENDS 2010 TO 2013

According to CMS, 2,217 hospitals were penalized an estimated $280 million in the initial year of the penalty program, increasing slightly to 2,225 hospitals in the program's second year (Rau 2013). After readmission rates held steady above 19 percent for several years, at the end of 2012 the Obama administration reported that hospital readmission rates had fallen to 17.2 percent. This news was encouraging because it amounted to 70,000 fewer unnecessary readmissions in the first year of the program and 130,000 fewer in the second year (Daly 2013). Furthermore, the reduction was a welcome development because readmission rates had largely held steady since the penalty was announced in 2010.

An interesting side note is that rural and critical access hospitals showed the largest readmission improvements in these initial measurement years. According to a study of 450 hospitals by the Premier Healthcare Alliance, rural hospitals showed an 11.2 percent drop in readmissions compared with a 10.2 percent reduction among other hospital groups (Daly 2013).

TACTICAL APPROACHES TO THE READMISSION PROBLEM

Though this chapter contains a great deal of statistics and data, this information is necessary to help you determine how to approach the readmission problem in your facility. The rest of this book will be light on data and quantification and more focused on tactical approaches to preventing unnecessary readmissions.

Again, as you read this book, I encourage you to grab a marker, highlight each tactical approach that might work in your organization, and add it to a list you can review when you have finished reading. Now that you know how the problem came to be, the fun part is determining how to address it and return to providing value-based care and preventing unnecessary readmissions. Enjoy!

REFERENCES

Abrams, M., and M. Levy. 2013. "Diagnosing and Treating Readmissions." *Hospital and Health Networks Daily.* Published January. www.hhnmag.com/display/HHN-news-article .dhtml?dcrPath=/templatedata/HF_Common/NewsArticle /data/HHN/Daily/2013/Jan/abrams012913-1580005365.

Center for Medicare Advocacy (CMA). 2014. "Reducing Rehospitalizations . . . the Right Way." Accessed August 27. www.medicareadvocacy.org/reducing-rehospitalizations %e2%80%a6-the-right-way/.

Centers for Medicare & Medicaid Services (CMS). 2014. "National Medicare Readmission Findings: Recent Data and Trends." Accessed December 18. www.academyhealth.org /files/2012/sunday/brennan.pdf.

Daly, R. 2013. "Reform Is Curbing Readmissions, CMS Says." *Modern Healthcare.* Published February 28. www.modern healthcare.com/article/20130228/NEWS/302289969.

Elixhauser, A., D. H. Au, and J. Podulka. 2011. "Readmissions for Chronic Obstructive Pulmonary Disease, 2008." Agency for Healthcare Research and Quality, Healthcare Cost and Utilization Project, Statistical Brief #121. Published September. www.hcup-us.ahrq.gov/reports/statbriefs/sb121.pdf.

Federal Register. 2013. "Part II—Department of Health and Human Services." 42 CFR Parts 412, 413, 414. Published August 19. www.gpo.gov/fdsys/pkg/FR-2013-08-19/pdf /2013-18956.pdf.

Khan, F. 2013. "Reducing Hospital Readmissions Rates: How to Avoid Upcoming Penalties and Maintain Patient Wellness." *Becker's Hospital Review.* Published December 17. www .beckershospitalreview.com/quality/reducing-hospital -readmissions-rates-how-to-avoid-upcoming-penalties-and -maintain-patient-wellness.html.

Patient Protection and Affordable Care Act (ACA). 2010. Pub. L. No. 111-148, 125 Stat. 119. www.gpo.gov/fdsys/pkg /PLAW-111publ148/pdf/PLAW-111publ148.pdf.

Qasim, M., and R. M. Andrews. 2012. "Post-surgical Readmissions Among Patients Living in the Poorest Communities, 2009." Agency for Healthcare Research and Quality, Healthcare Cost and Utilization Project, Statistical Brief #142. Published September. www.hcup-us.ahrq.gov /reports/statbriefs/sb142.pdf.

Rau, J. 2013. "Rehospitalization Rates Fell in First Year of Medicare Penalties." *Kaiser Health News.* Published December 9. http://capsules.kaiserhealthnews.org/index.php/2013/12 /rehospitalization-rates-fell-in-first-year-of-medicare-penalties/.

Rizzo, E. 2013. "6 Stats on the Cost of Readmissions for CMS-Tracked Conditions." *Becker's Hospital Review.* Published December 12. www.beckershospitalreview.com/quality /6-stats-on-the-cost-of-readmission-for-cms-tracked -conditions.html.

CHAPTER 2

Moving Beyond the Gold Standard

As we work together to prevent readmissions, one of the biggest challenges is the traditional perspective of hospital C-suite executives. For more than 30 years, talented, experienced hospital leaders have understandably been focused on doing one thing and one thing only: putting heads in beds.

THE "PUTTING HEADS IN BEDS" MIND-SET

Most seasoned hospital and health system executives have spent their career focused on two primary tactics to drive volume and ensure a consistent inpatient census: (1) marketing to high-volume physicians to capture market share and (2) building inpatient specialty programs to drive inpatient volume. Other traditional tactics to drive acute care volume include contracting with key managed care partners and aligning with post-acute care providers to ensure that yours is the facility of choice when patients need acute care. The reality is that hospitals still only get paid when a head is in a bed. Creative risk arrangements, accountable care organizations

(ACOs), and bundled-payment initiative programs exist, but no one is getting rich from Medicare Shared Savings Plan ACO bonuses. In fact, it remains challenging to turn a profit in the hospital environment (even in an ACO program).

After so many years of putting all their energy toward driving inpatient census to build revenue, these seasoned executives are not likely to make proactive moves to prevent readmissions. They do not perceive the readmission penalty as a significant threat. Furthermore, implementing tactics to prevent readmissions is contrary to every tactic they have ever used to ensure success and profitability in the past. I once heard a seasoned healthcare executive state, "Even in an era where we are reimbursed based on value, inpatient census remains the 'gold standard' for hospital revenue." The gold standard. "That's it," I thought. "The gold standard is the obstacle the rest of the healthcare continuum faces when discussing the readmission issue with seasoned hospital executives."

In 2013, as I began to do research for this book, my goal was to learn as much as I could about care coordination and readmissions prevention and to identify all of the existing solutions. One thing I heard from the vendors and solution providers who were marketing to hospitals to prevent readmissions was the resistance they experienced from C-suite executives. Why? Well, because of the gold standard, of course. A seasoned C-suite executive will gladly listen to proposals that will bring value and increased revenue to his organization, but proposals that only reduce costs are much tougher to sell. Changing this mind-set is a goal of this book.

THE PROBLEM OF OBSERVATION DAYS

A bigger issue for current health system executives is how to manage and handle the growing problem of observation census. *Observation status* is a term hospitals use when an emergency department physician is not able to justify an inpatient admission but is not comfortable discharging the patient home. The patient is often placed in a "holding bed"—that is, a hospital bed outside the emergency department—and observed for several hours to determine the need and justification for inpatient admission. The federal government reimburses for observation at outpatient rates, which are about 80 to 90 percent lower than inpatient reimbursement. The hospital's costs for caring for observation patients is similar to their costs for caring for inpatients, however, so observation status wreaks financial havoc on hospital cost-management efforts.

The single most critical issue for hospitals in 2013 was the Medicare Recovery Audit Program, and the end result of those audits was a significant increase in observation days. Although the Recovery Audit Program was put on hold in 2014, it did not go away entirely. The federal government used these audits to take back billions of Medicare dollars from hospitals for patients whose charts lacked adequate documentation to justify an acute care stay. In addition, 2013 brought a trend of managed care organizations attempting to stage patients on hospital observation units as a means of reducing expenses.

Although 2013 brought a welcome decrease in unnecessary hospital readmissions nationwide (Daly 2013), the increase in observation days suggests that putting patients on observation units is one way hospitals are approaching the readmission issue. Several studies have illustrated that the increase in observation days was nearly equivalent to the decrease in readmitted patient days (Carlson 2013).

Observation days and the accompanying reimbursement issues pertaining to observation status are a problem that will not be solved in the near future. Although hospitals and health systems can use observation units as a tactic to help reduce readmissions, it is one of the most costly tactics to avoid the readmission penalty. Chapter 5, "Prevention Planning Phase Three: The Patient Returns to the Emergency Department," provides greater detail on when observation units can be an appropriate solution to prevent readmissions.

COLLECTING READMISSION DATA

The other issue hospitals have been slow to address is the need to collect readmission data on their own hospital. Most hospitals know little about their readmission rate, let alone what is driving it. Although some hospitals have made readmission prevention a priority, they remain in the minority. The time has come for the healthcare community to change that and develop effective systems to prevent unnecessary hospital admissions.

Hospitals can access significant detail on their hospital-specific readmission rates with little effort. The Centers for Medicare & Medicaid Services (CMS) requires quality improvement organizations to distribute regular readmission reports, and these reports are not only specific to the five diagnosis categories in the readmission penalty but also go into great detail to show how each hospital is affected by readmissions from skilled-nursing facilities (SNFs), home health agencies, and other post-acute care entities. Other sources that provide readmission data include Medicare Compare (www .medicare.gov), Kaiser Health News (www.kaiserhealthnews.com), No Place Like Home (www.noplacelikehomeaz.org), the National Readmission Prevention Collaborative (www.nationalreadmission prevention.com), the CMS-distributed Program for Evaluating Payment Patterns Electronic Reports (PEPPERs), and acute care facility–based programs such as Crimson.

Some of the solutions discussed in this book provide real-time readmission data for hospitals that are not willing to wait for the often-outdated data provided on those websites, however. RightCare Solutions, developed by Dr. Kathryn Bowles at the University of Pennsylvania School of Nursing, for example, offers a product that identifies disease-specific and SNF-specific readmission rates for hospitals. COMS Interactive, developed by a physician and his son (a nursing home administrator), is a predictive software that breaks down disease-specific readmission rates for SNFs and assisted-living communities in real time.

If an organization is not reviewing and sharing these data regularly—quarterly, at a minimum—it is not prioritizing the readmission penalty or taking it seriously. Hospitals that seek solutions and strive to coordinate care in their community not only make internal efforts to gather data from their existing software system but also reach out to their post-acute care providers to share the data they collect. Although the organizations making these efforts are still in the minority, by sharing best practices they are slowly educating themselves on the intricacies of the readmission issue in their specific community and how to best address it. The Perspective at the end of this chapter describes how proper documentation and coding of conditions defining the readmissions cohort can support effective case management strategies.

NO COOKIE-CUTTER ANSWERS

The readmission issue is specific to each community and its unique providers, and this book will illustrate that there is no cookie-cutter, one-size-fits-all readmission prevention plan that works for everyone. In fact, this book was written for the exact opposite purpose. Each community needs to develop a readmission prevention plan specific to its needs. By sharing the tactics in this book and discussing best-practice case studies, each community can pick and choose the tactics that will work for its hospital and post-acute care providers to prevent unnecessary readmissions.

One of the first lessons this book will share is that the hospitals and health systems that are taking the readmission and care coordination issue seriously have found that there is no such thing as too much readmissions data. Hospitals that are looking at the readmission data from every angle are learning more and more as each month passes. Although the issue of readmission prevention may still be in its infancy, hospitals are currently in the fourth year of the penalty phase, and additional penalties and incentives for improved care coordination will continue to be introduced through the Affordable

Care Act (ACA) into 2018. Those penalties may have been insignificant in the eyes of many hospital executives, but the accumulation of the ACA's penalties and incentives to coordinate care will eventually be too important for hospital executives to continue to ignore.

Care coordination is here. It is real, it cannot be avoided, and it is time to address it. One of the most effective ways to coordinate care and bring post-acute care providers together is by approaching the readmission prevention issue as a collaborative team. This book discusses and illustrates a variety of tactics that can be considered by any individual or team planning to implement a hospital-specific or community-specific readmission prevention program.

PERSPECTIVE

The Impact of ICD-9-CM and ICD-10 on Readmission Measurement Under the ACA

By James S. Kennedy, MD
President, CDIMD Physician Champions

The Medicare Payment Advisory Commission's (MedPAC) 2008 *Report to the Congress: Reforming the Delivery System* recommended that federal health programs measure and publish individual hospital readmission rates. But even before that report, the Centers for Medicare & Medicaid Services (CMS) and various state Medicaid programs had been strategically developing and honing tools that measure readmission rates and their financial impact. The MedPAC report estimated that Medicare's expenditures for potentially preventable readmissions might be as high as $12 billion per year. A 2009 study funded by the Institute for Healthcare Improvement and the John A. Hartford Foundation estimated that almost one-fifth (19.6 percent) of the 11,855,702 Medicare beneficiaries who were discharged from a hospital in 2003–2004 were rehospitalized within 30 days, and 34 percent were rehospitalized within 90 days, costing the Medicare system $17.2 billion in 2004 (Jencks,

→

Williams, and Coleman 2009). Readmission reduction is also emphasized in the Affordable Care Act (ACA).

Many readmission studies and findings are derived from an analysis of inpatient hospital insurance claims that are risk adjusted using patient characteristics derived from submitted International Classification of Diseases, Ninth Revision, Clinical Modification (ICD-9-CM) codes or, after October 1, 2015, the Tenth Revision ICD-10-CM codes. As a result, CMS and other analysts use these administrative claims data to measure readmission rates and offer incentives for their reduction.

Current algorithms include the following:

- *CMS Hospital Admissions Reduction Program*: Through this program, authorized by the ACA and the Social Security Act, CMS (2014) uses the index admission's ICD-9-CM codes and all codes for the previous year to identify measured cohorts and to estimate the likelihood that a readmission will occur. Developed by Yale University researchers under contract with CMS, the tool is in the public domain and available for public review (www.quality net.org). An ICD-10 version is not publicly available.
- *Medicare Spending per Beneficiary (MSPB)*: Although not a direct measure of readmissions, MSPB measures the risk-adjusted cost of hospital care within a period of 3 days before admission to 30 days after admission, which includes any readmissions. To account for case-mix variation and other factors, the MSPB methodology also adjusts for age and severity of illness. This model broadly follows the CMS Hierarchical Condition Categories (HCC) methodology used by Medicare Advantage plans, which is derived from the ICD-9-CM codes taken from the beneficiary's Medicare Part A and Part B claims during the 90-day period before the start of the episode;

$\rightarrow$

it is an indicator of whether the beneficiary recently required long-term care and includes the Medicare Severity Diagnosis-Related Group (DRG) (also ICD-9-CM based) of the index hospitalization. The MSPB affects both the CMS physician and hospital value-based payment calculations. A description of the MSPB is available on the CMS website (www.qualitynet.org).

◆ *3M's Potentially Preventable Readmissions (PPR) Grouping Software*: 3M Health Information Systems (3MHIS), a subsidiary of the 3M Corporation, developed its own proprietary readmissions algorithm using ICD-9-CM codes (www.3MHIS.com). Texas, Maryland, and Illinois are among the many states analyzing claims data with the PPR algorithm and are either publishing their findings on state-supported websites or incentivizing state-governed reimbursements on the basis of provider performance. A PPR definitions manual based on the ICD-9-CM is available for purchase from 3MHIS, or a representative sample may be downloaded using information available on various state-sanctioned websites. An ICD-10 PPR definitions manual is available only to licensed subscribers through the 3MHIS website.

◆ Other readmissions tools based on ICD-9-CM codes exist and are used by governments, payers, and providers to measure and influence behaviors. These include

- University HealthSystem Consortium (UHC) (www.uhc .edu), which is available only to UHC members;

- The Pennsylvania Health Care Cost Containment Council (www.phc4.org);

- Comparion Analytics (http://comparionanalytics.com /risk-adjustment-methods/), a proprietary product that requires a relationship with Comparion for access;

- Truven Analytics (www.truvenhealth.com), a proprietary product that requires a relationship with Truven for access; and

$\rightarrow$

- California Office of Statewide Health Planning and Development (http://oshpd.ca.gov).

A review of some aspects of these tools will show how the provider documentation and ICD-9-CM code assignment affects readmission rate calculation and suggests a course of action to ensure their integrity before claim submission as part of a facility's overall readmission management strategy.

How Inpatient Facility Claims Data Affect the Reported Readmission Rate

Most readmissions tools calculate their findings as a ratio of the observed (actual) readmission rate to the expected (predicted) readmission rate, commonly known as the O/E ratio. Expressed in another way,

$$\text{Risk-adjusted readmission rate} = \frac{\text{Observed readmission rate for the defined cohort}}{\text{Expected readmission rate for the defined cohort}}$$

Given that the risk-adjusted readmission rate is a ratio, it can be reduced or favorably influenced by ascertaining whether the cohort being measured is properly described by the provider's documentation and whether the submitted and sequenced ICD-9-CM codes (e.g., pneumonia, heart failure) applicable to the condition being measured are clinically congruent; documenting and coding all conditions or procedures that would exclude the case from the cohort; lowering the actual observed readmission rate for the defined cohort through effective case management; or increasing the expected readmission rate by ensuring that all appropriate ICD-9-CM codes involved in the risk-adjustment variables affecting this metric are captured. Not uncommonly, a measured risk-adjusted readmission rate is artificially high because the condition(s) excluding the case from being assigned to the cohort and/or the comorbidities defining the severity of the expected readmission rate were not

$\longrightarrow$

documented by the provider, were not coded or properly sequenced by the facility when reported, or both. This can happen even though effective case management strategies that are discussed elsewhere in this book and that favorably affect the observed rate have been implemented.

Specific Elements of Hospital Data Affecting Cohort Selection and Risk Adjustment

Data for each hospital encounter are submitted electronically using ASC X12N 837 version 5010 software or on paper using the UB-04 universal claim form. Data elements are assigned by different departments on the basis of explicit medical record documentation or through patient interviews. The following sections describe elements that affect cohort selection or readmission rate calculations.

Primary or Secondary Insurance

CMS's inpatient value-based purchasing program for readmissions applies only to traditional Medicare, not Medicare Advantage, programs. If a readmission rate is being calculated by a particular payer, such as traditional Medicare, the readmission will count only if the patient is identified as having traditional Medicare. In certain circumstances, traditional Medicare should not be billed for an inpatient admission, such as for a noncovered cosmetic procedure. Providers must ensure the integrity of each patient's insurance information for each encounter and follow their negotiated contracts and rules for claim submission.

Discharge Status Codes

Although many tools count all readmissions within a certain time frame, such as 30 or 60 days, some exclude planned readmissions if they are identified as such on the index

→

admission. Effective October 1, 2013, the National Uniform Billing Committee added new discharge status codes that report if a readmission is planned (see Exhibit 2.1).

Exhibit 2.1 New Discharge Status Codes

Base Code	New Code	Discharge Status Code Title
01	81	Discharged to Home or Self-Care with a Planned Acute Care Hospital Inpatient Readmission
02	82	Discharged/Transferred to a Short-Term General Hospital for Inpatient Care with a Planned Acute Care Hospital Inpatient Readmission
03	83	Discharged/Transferred to a Skilled Nursing Facility (SNF) with Medicare Certification with a Planned Acute Care Hospital Inpatient Readmission
04	84	Discharged/Transferred to a Facility That Provides Custodial or Supportive Care with a Planned Acute Care Hospital Inpatient Readmission
05	85	Discharged/Transferred to a Designated Cancer Center or Children's Hospital with a Planned Acute Care Hospital Inpatient Readmission
06	86	Discharged/Transferred to Home Under Care of Organized Home Health Service Organization with a Planned Acute Care Hospital Inpatient Readmission

(continued)

→

21	87	Discharged/Transferred to Court/Law Enforcement with a Planned Acute Care Hospital Inpatient Readmission
43	88	Discharged/Transferred to a Federal Health Care Facility with a Planned Acute Care Hospital Inpatient Readmission
61	89	Discharged/Transferred to a Hospital-Based Medicare Approved Swing Bed with a Planned Acute Care Hospital Inpatient Readmission
62	90	Discharged/Transferred to an Inpatient Rehabilitation Facility (IRF) Including Rehabilitation Distinct Part Units of a Hospital with a Planned Acute Care Hospital Inpatient Readmission
63	91	Discharged/Transferred to a Medicare Certified Long-Term Care Hospital (LTCH) with a Planned Acute Care Hospital Inpatient Readmission
64	92	Discharged/Transferred to a Nursing Facility Certified Under Medicaid but Not Certified Under Medicare with a Planned Acute Care Hospital Inpatient Readmission
65	93	Discharged/Transferred to a Psychiatric Hospital or Psychiatric Distinct Part Unit of a Hospital with a Planned Acute Care Hospital Inpatient Readmission
66	94	Discharged/Transferred to a Critical Access Hospital (CAR) with a Planned Acute Care Hospital Inpatient Readmission
70	95	Discharged/Transferred to Another Type of Health Care Institution Not Defined Elsewhere in This Code List with a Planned Acute Care Hospital Inpatient Readmission

Source: 78 Fed. Reg. 160 (Aug. 19, 2013), 50539.

→

If it is known at the time of discharge that a readmission is planned, then this must be clearly documented in a location where the person assigning the discharge status code (usually an abstractor in health information management) can clearly see and assign it. Although these cases may not affect all readmission tools currently in place, their complete and accurate capture provides policymakers with the data needed to revise current readmission tools if necessary. In a similar manner, index admissions where the discharge status code signifies that the patient left against medical advice or transferred to another acute care facility often disqualify the admission as an index admission for the readmissions tool.

Principal Diagnosis

Defined in the Uniform Hospital Discharge Data Set and the ICD-9-CM Official Guidelines for Coding and Reporting as "that condition *established after study* to be *chiefly* responsible for occasioning the [inpatient] admission of the patient to the hospital for care" [emphasis added], the principal diagnosis often determines whether the admission will serve as the index encounter for a particular cohort (e.g., pneumonia, heart failure, myocardial infarction) in which a readmission after a certain period of time (e.g., 30 days) will count toward a penalty. The principal diagnosis is usually assigned by the facility's inpatient coding department on the basis of provider documentation and sequencing rules governed by ICD-9-CM, its official guidelines, and official advice published in the American Hospital Association's *Coding Clinic for ICD-9-CM.* An erroneous or clinically incongruent principal diagnosis assignment could mislabel an inpatient admission as an index encounter for which a readmission could count toward a penalty. Following are some examples of how the principal diagnoses of pneumonia, congestive heart failure, and chronic obstructive pulmonary disease (COPD) are handled.

→

Pneumonia

In the CMS Hospital Admissions Reduction Program developed by Yale University, an index admission governing the pneumonia metric requires a principal diagnosis of various pneumonia codes (see Exhibit 2.2).

Exhibit 2.2 The ICD-9-CM Codes Defining Pneumonia

- ◆ 480.0 Pneumonia due to adenovirus
- ◆ 480.1 Pneumonia due to respiratory syncytial virus
- ◆ 480.2 Pneumonia due to parainfluenza virus
- ◆ 480.3 Pneumonia due to SARS-associated coronavirus
- ◆ 480.8 Viral pneumonia: pneumonia due to other virus not elsewhere classified
- ◆ 480.9 Viral pneumonia unspecified
- ◆ 481.0 Pneumococcal pneumonia (*Streptococcus pneumoniae* pneumonia)
- ◆ 482.0 Pneumonia due to *Klebsiella pneumoniae*
- ◆ 482.1 Pneumonia due to *Pseudomonas*
- ◆ 482.2 Pneumonia due to *Haemophilus influenzae*
- ◆ 482.3 Pneumonia due to *Streptococcus* unspecified
- ◆ 482.31 Pneumonia due to *Streptococcus* group A
- ◆ 482.32 Pneumonia due to *Streptococcus* group B
- ◆ 482.39 Pneumonia due to other *Streptococcus*
- ◆ 482.4 Pneumonia due to *Staphylococcus* unspecified
- ◆ 482.41 Pneumonia due to *Staphylococcus aureus*
- ◆ 482.42 Methicillin-resistant pneumonia due to *Staphylococcus aureus*
- ◆ 482.49 Other *Staphylococcus* pneumonia
- ◆ 482.81 Pneumonia due to anaerobes
- ◆ 482.82 Pneumonia due to *Escherichia coli*
- ◆ 482.83 Pneumonia due to other gram-negative bacteria
- ◆ 482.84 Pneumonia due to Legionnaires' disease
- ◆ 482.89 Pneumonia due to other specified bacteria

→

- 482.9 Bacterial pneumonia unspecified
- 483.0 Pneumonia due to *Mycoplasma pneumoniae*
- 483.1 Pneumonia due to chlamydia
- 483.8 Pneumonia due to other specified organism
- 485.0 Bronchopneumonia organism unspecified
- 486.0 Pneumonia organism unspecified
- 487.0 Influenza with pneumonia
- 488.11 Influenza due to identified novel H1N1 influenza virus with pneumonia

Source: Adapted from Krumholz et al. (2008).

Note that aspiration pneumonia, sepsis, and acute respiratory failure that is present on admission and qualifying as a principal diagnosis are not on the list; thus, if these conditions are present, documented, and compliantly sequenced as the principal diagnosis, the inpatient encounter will not count as an index admission for the CMS pneumonia readmission methodology. In other words, if a patient is admitted with pneumonia on the index admission but also meets the clinical criteria for sepsis due to pneumonia (e.g., toxic appearance, white blood cell count above 12,000, temperature above 101°F, tachycardia, and/or tachypnea that is not due to another condition) and is documented as having sepsis due to pneumonia at the time of admission and optimally again in the discharge summary, the encounter is not included as an index admission for CMS's pneumonia readmission tool if the coder sequences sepsis as the principal diagnosis. If the physician fails to document sepsis due to pneumonia on admission (even though the patient had the condition), a pneumonia diagnosis will be sequenced as the principal diagnosis, assigning the admission to the pneumonia readmission cohort. Documented aspiration pneumonia treated with reasonable antibiotics (e.g., clindamycin, metronidazole, Zosyn®, or higher-dose $\rightarrow$

levofloxacin) and coded as the principal diagnosis likewise does not count as an index admission, whereas a commonly used synonym, "healthcare-associated pneumonia," does. The same can be said for any other condition coexisting with pneumonia as a reason for inpatient admission; if the alternative condition is documented, coded, and sequenced as the principal diagnosis, the admission does not count as an index admission in CMS's pneumonia readmission algorithm, though it may qualify for another cohort.

Congestive heart failure

As with pneumonia, CMS uses various ICD-9-CM codes for heart failure sequenced as the principal diagnosis to qualify the inpatient encounter as the index admission for its heart failure readmission tool. If a patient is admitted with congestive heart failure but acute respiratory failure is present on admission (e.g., in the emergency department) and factored into the decision to admit the patient as an inpatient, the patient's acute respiratory failure excludes that admission as an index admission for the CMS heart failure readmissions tool if it is documented as such and sequenced as the principal diagnosis.

Another example relates to troponin elevations that are commonly present in patients admitted with decompensated heart failure. Research has shown that an elevated troponin level in a patient with acute heart failure is predictive of death, so providers and facilities must ensure that those cases are properly classified (Peacock et al. 2008). Therefore, if a patient admitted with heart failure has symptoms or signs of acute myocardial ischemia and a new increase or decrease in serum troponin levels at the 99th upper reference limit (usually around 0.1 ng/mL), definition and documentation that the

→

patient's heart failure exacerbation was associated with an acute myocardial infarction and sequencing the myocardial infarction code as the principal diagnosis reclassifies the admission from the heart failure cohort to the acute myocardial infarction cohort, one with a higher expected and more clinically congruent readmission rate.

In a different vein, if a patient with chronic cor pulmonale due to COPD is admitted with anasarca and the provider states that the final diagnosis was decompensated isolated right heart failure, ICD-9-CM classifies this as unspecified or biventricular heart failure, which, if sequenced as the principal diagnosis, is an index admission for the heart failure cohort, not the COPD cohort. Whether a code for cor pulmonale should be sequenced as a principal diagnosis depends on the provider's documentation (especially in the discharge summary) and the coding department's view on assigning and sequencing these codes, given that ICD-9-CM (and ICD-10) and the *Coding Clinic for ICD-9-CM* have conflicting advice on how to manage these admissions.

Chronic obstructive pulmonary disease

In this methodology, various ICD-9-CM codes for COPD sequenced as the principal diagnosis or acute respiratory failure sequenced as the principal diagnosis with a COPD-related code sequenced as a secondary diagnosis qualifies the admission for the COPD cohort. Asthma without COPD as a principal diagnosis does not qualify a case as an index admission, yet some providers are not precise with their language and might label an asthma case as chronic obstructive asthma, thus qualifying the case as COPD, even if it does not meet the clinical criteria.

$\rightarrow$

Other cohorts or tools

The definitions manuals for each tool should be consulted
to learn which ICD-9-CM code includes or excludes an
admission from a particular cohort. For example, 3M's PPR
methodology allows for "rerouting" of certain secondary
diagnoses to define cohorts rather than relying solely on
the principal diagnosis. As an example, if a child with cystic
fibrosis is admitted with pneumonia as a principal diagnosis,
3M reroutes the secondary diagnosis of cystic fibrosis to
place the child's admission in the cystic fibrosis DRG, not a
pneumonia DRG. Psychiatric diagnoses or admissions for
treatment of cancer as the principal diagnosis exclude an
admission from CMS's Hospital-Wide All-Cause Unplanned
Readmission tool.

Essentials for principal diagnosis assignment

A rigorous clinical documentation and coding integrity
process bridging the gap between the provider and coder
is essential to ascertain that the principal diagnosis
properly describes the reason for the patient's inpatient
admission, is supported by the clinical circumstances,
and is correctly assigned by the coding department. If
the circumstances of admission, diagnostic approach,
or treatment rendered are not completely or consistently
documented by a provider in the language required by
ICD-9-CM, a provider query to clarify these circumstances
is suggested before ICD-9-CM code assignment.
Case management, quality, coding, and compliance
departments, along with executive leadership, can
facilitate physician engagement with open communication
regarding ICD-9-CM coding rules and how they affect their
own CMS value-based payment modifiers.

→

Secondary Diagnoses

The 5010 electronic transaction set allows up to 24 additional diagnosis codes to be assigned for an inpatient admission. In all risk-adjustment tools, the quantity and quality of these codes influence the expected readmission rate, given that certain codes are more heavily weighted to predicting the readmission than others. For example, in the CMS Yale University model, a documented and coded diagnosis of sleep apnea, respiratory failure, heart failure, and shock, among other conditions documented within the previous year, increases the expected readmission rate. Other conditions that are commonly not documented (though known to the physician) include malnutrition (not just low body mass index), functional quadriplegia (not bed confinement status), hemiparesis (not right- or left-sided weakness), and various anemias. A documented diagnosis and ICD-9-CM code of morbid obesity affect the expected readmission rate for total joint replacement; a code for simple obesity or body mass index greater than 40 does not. A list of ICD-9-CM codes qualifying for the expected readmission risk-adjustment variables is available on the QualityNet website (www.qualitynet.org).

The 3M PPR model uses more diagnoses, which are grouped into its All-Payer-Refined Diagnosis-Related Group (APR-DRG) Severity of Illness (SOI) models, which are described in the definitions manuals previously referenced. 3M classifies the SOI into four tiers based on the submitted ICD-9-CM codes and to some extent the patient's age or procedures, with Level 1 being the lowest and Level 4 being the highest. Hospitals must license an APR-DRG grouper to calculate the APR-DRG SOI and learn the effect of each diagnosis, optimally before the patient's code submission, so as to determine the need for a second review

→

identifying incomplete, imprecise, or clinically incongruent documentation. Again, as with principal diagnosis assignment, clinical documentation and coding integrity are crucial to proper readmission risk adjustment for the secondary diagnoses.

Outpatient Claims Data

Unlike most inpatient readmissions tools that rely only on the inpatient claim for risk adjustment (e.g., the 3M PPR or UHC models), CMS uses outpatient claims submitted within 12 months of the index admission to capture diagnoses calculating the expected readmission rate, particularly with the Yale readmissions model applicable to the hospital value-based payment and the HCCs for the MSPB methodology. Although the outpatient or physician electronic billing standard allows for only 12 diagnoses to be submitted for each encounter, given that patients usually have multiple encounters with different providers within a year of an index admission for the Yale model and six months for the HCC model, the expected readmission risk may be optimized by ensuring the completeness and integrity of outpatient diagnosis code submission before the index admission. Consequently, many facilities (particularly SNFs, which will soon be judged by their own readmissions metrics, and hospitals affected by the CMS readmissions rates) are emphasizing integrity of clinical documentation and coding integrity for outpatient claims submitted by their employed or referring physicians, given that CMS uses these to predict a potential readmission (American Health Care Association 2014a, 2014b).

Summary

If one is to have any chance of winning a game, one must know the rules and how to keep score. Although effective

$\rightarrow$

case management strategies described elsewhere in this book are crucial to success in reducing actual or observed readmissions, unless the documentation and coding of conditions defining the readmissions cohort (the observed metric) and determining the expected readmissions rate are properly vetted and maintained, the O/E ratio by which readmission rates are calculated can be compromised. Forming partnerships with physician leaders, coders, and case management and compliance departments in promoting clinical documentation and coding integrity in compliance with the provider's clinical intent and the ICD-9-CM or ICD-10 code assignment conventions is an integral part of managing inpatient readmissions and improving patient outcomes.

REFERENCES

American Health Care Association. 2014a. "Reducing Hospital Readmissions: Skilled Nursing Facility Value-Based Purchasing Program." Accessed June 25. www.ahcancal.org /advocacy/solutions/Pages/HospitalReadmissions.aspx.

———. 2014b. "Skilled Nursing Facility Value-Based Purchasing Program: A Hospital Readmissions Reduction Program for SNFs." Issue brief. Published April 5. www.ahcancal.org /advocacy/solutions/Documents/Value%20Based%20 Purchasing%20-%20IB.PDF.

Carlson, J. 2013. "Faulty Gauge? Readmission Rates Are Down, but Observational-Status Patients Are Up—and That Could Skew Medicare Numbers." *Modern Healthcare*. Published June 8. www.modernhealthcare.com/article/20130608 /MAGAZINE/306089991.

Centers for Medicare & Medicaid Services (CMS). 2014. "Readmissions Reduction Program." Accessed June 24. www.cms.gov/Medicare/Medicare-Fee-for-Service-Payment /AcuteInpatientPPS/Readmissions-Reduction-Program.html.

Daly, R. 2013. "Reform Is Curbing Readmissions, CMS Says." *Modern Healthcare*. Published February 28. www.modern healthcare.com/article/20130228/NEWS/302289969 /reform-is-curbing-readmissions-cms-says.

Jencks, S. F., M. V. Williams, and E. A. Coleman. 2009. "Rehospitalizations Among Patients in the Medicare Fee for Service Program." *New England Journal of Medicine* 360 (14): 1418–28. Accessed June 24, 2014. www.nejm.org/doi/full /10.1056/NEJMsa0803563.

Krumholz, H. M., S.-L. T. Normand, P. S. Keenan, M. M. Desai, Z. Lin, E. E. Drye, K. R. Bhat, and G. C. Schreiner. 2008. *Hospital 30-Day Pneumonia Readmission Measure*. New Haven, CT: Yale University/Yale-New Haven Hospital Center for Outcomes Research & Evaluation.

Medicare Payment Advisory Commission (MedPAC). 2008. *Report to the Congress: Reforming the Delivery System*. Accessed June 24, 2014. http://medpac.gov/documents/reports/Jun08 _EntireReport.pdf?sfvrsn=0.

Peacock, W. F., T. De Marco, G. C. Fonarow, D. Diercks, J. Wynne, F. S. Apple, and A. H. B. Wu for the ADHERE Investigators. 2008. "Cardiac Troponin and Outcome in Acute Heart Failure." *New England Journal of Medicine* 358 (20): 2117–26. Accessed September 23, 2014. www.nejm .org/doi/full/10.1056/NEJMoa0706824.

Part II

THE THREE PHASES
OF PREPARATION TO
PREVENT READMISSIONS

CHAPTER 3

Prevention Planning Phase One: Before Discharge

The goal of this book is to provide specific readmission prevention solutions for healthcare operators. To provide a clear understanding of each tactic, readmission prevention planning has been divided into three phases:

- Phase One: Before discharge
- Phase Two: After discharge
- Phase Three: When the patient returns to the emergency department

Mapping solutions to these three points in the care continuum provides an efficient way for acute and post-acute care providers to identify specific tactics that may be worth implementing in their community and in their organization.

To review, the readmission penalties implemented by the Centers for Medicare & Medicaid Services (CMS) apply to Medicare fee-for-service patients (in five disease categories: acute myocardial infarction, congestive heart failure, pneumonia, chronic obstructive pulmonary disease, and joint replacement) who are readmitted to any short-term acute care hospital for any reason within 30 days of being discharged from a hospital. In short, the discharging hospital is penalized when a patient is readmitted to any hospital within 30 days of the discharge date of the index stay.

Planned readmissions (such as surgeries and other scheduled procedures) are not subject to the penalty, and CMS has provided (via the *Federal Register*) additional codes and information on how to plan for and document them. However, more work must be done to aggregate the data to determine which readmissions should be subject to readmission penalties as a result of hospitals not appropriately coordinating care.

Phase One focuses on information that can be gathered while the patient is still in the hospital and includes tactics the hospital and care team can deploy before the patient is discharged from the initial hospital stay (the index stay). Such data can help the facility more accurately predict patients' likelihood of being readmitted on the basis of their overall health and care plan. Other Phase One tactics focus on implementing organizational changes to prevent readmissions and collecting facility-specific information that will help the organization identify potential readmission problems. Recommended Phase One tactics are described in detail in the rest of the chapter.

CONDUCT PATIENT RISK ASSESSMENTS

The most important thing hospitals can do to prevent unnecessary readmissions and thus avoid the readmission penalty is capture as much data as possible about the patient at each patient encounter. The integration of electronic health records in the hospital and the physician's office is making that task easier.

The most common form of data gathering during the index stay relates to risk assessment. Once relevant patient information is collected, the hospital then uses a risk assessment tool to interpret the data. Data collected include information gathered from the patient, family, friend, or medical professional when the patient arrived at the hospital; any available medical history (stored within the hospital's medical records or provided by the patient and/or family); demographic information; and multiple social determinants if available, including current living situation (home or facility), access to transportation, care providers, and food and hydration sources. Each of these factors has proven to be relevant in determining a patient's likelihood to be readmitted to the hospital.

Hospitals use different methods of conducting risk assessments. Many use nurses or other employees to conduct risk assessment by hand, but a number of software packages are now available that perform risk stratification on patients and will likely become the norm as hospitals begin to prioritize and set aside funds for population management efforts. Regardless of the method by which a hospital or health system conducts a risk assessment, it is critical that patients who are at high risk to return to the hospital be identified as soon as possible.

At a March 2014 meeting in San Diego, Dawn Hohl, director of customer service at the Johns Hopkins Home Care Group, gave a presentation about the organization's successful Discharge Planning Team model using the case study of a patient who had been readmitted more than 20 times in one year. After identifying that this patient was a proven high risk for readmission, Johns Hopkins Medicine contacted the health plan to suggest a remote monitoring device that could be used in the patient's home. Because the patient had been such a heavy user of the hospital, the health plan agreed to pay for the remote monitoring device; as a result, the patient was not readmitted to the hospital in the next 12 months.

Many hospitals have implemented risk-stratification models that require significant input and documentation from hospitalists, attending physicians, nurses, and case managers. In most cases, risk-stratification models that rely on significant human data entry are not likely to be sustainable long term. Although some level of human input is necessary, solutions that seem to be gaining traction are those that can aggregate the necessary data electronically or with a brief questionnaire. A number of vendors have emerged as industry leaders in the sector, including RightCare Solutions, which took its risk-stratification product to market after extensive testing at the University of Pennsylvania Medical Center. Dr. Kathryn Bowles (2014), who championed the work, says that the entire solution is based on information collected during the initial emergency department visit.

Many other methods of conducting risk assessments are available to hospitals. Although this book does not go into detail on the process of risk stratification, an abundance of research is available on the topic, and software solutions are becoming affordable for hospitals. In the near future, risk stratification will become an almost completely automated process and will be one of the key components all hospitals will use to identify patients at high risk for readmission.

CREATE A POST-ACUTE CARE NETWORK

Establishing a coordinated post-acute care network of skilled-nursing facilities (SNFs) is another important tactic in preventing readmissions. The goal is to set an expectation for your post-acute care providers that encourages a commitment to quality, communication between providers, and collaboration to prevent readmissions.

Current CMS regulations require hospitals to add to their provider list every home health agency that submits a written request to be added. In urban areas such as Los Angeles, it is not uncommon for a hospital to have more than 100 home health agencies on its provider list. Similarly, federal regulations require hospitals to provide a complete list of local skilled-nursing providers, though it is up to the hospital to interpret the word "local." Hospitals have traditionally been hesitant to narrow their network of post-acute care providers because of these regulations, but the trend is changing as a result of the Affordable Care Act (ACA).

At least six initiatives in the ACA financially incentivize hospitals to coordinate care (see the Preface). To effectively coordinate care with post-acute care providers, however, hospitals realize that they must narrow their network of post-acute care providers and are finding that it can be difficult to coordinate work even with as few as three home health agencies. For this reason, in the coming years many hospitals and health systems will likely return to the home health business—even if it's simply a break-even proposition—in a reversal of the recent trend in which hospitals and health systems eliminated their home health agencies because they were not profitable. Hospitals and health systems will soon be burdened with the expense of multiple post-acute care products and services designed to prevent unnecessary readmissions. They will not be able to afford all of the needed solutions, so they will seek to establish new, non-traditional post-acute care product lines wherever possible, so long as they return even the smallest of margins.

Each hospital and health system uses its own set of criteria to identify who will be included in its narrow network. Quality care, longevity in the community, and proximity to the hospital and ancillary providers are all relevant factors. Hospitals should not feel obligated to identify criteria for the facilities that are included, however, nor should planning teams spend significant amounts of time worrying about the selection process.

The ACA mandates that hospitals coordinate care and penalizes hospitals if their partners provide substandard care. That's all the justification you need to narrow your network. However, if anyone is questioned about selection criteria, a standard answer would be "These are the providers who agreed to our criteria and with whom we came to an agreement when we began the initiative." See how easy that was? No attorneys needed. I have seen many a client and hospital system get stuck on this issue unnecessarily. I would argue that those who get stuck on how they can legally narrow their post-acute care network are living in a fee-for-service mentality. (Newsflash: Fee for service is history.)

Some hospitals also invite home health and hospice providers to their post-acute care network meetings. In my experience, when a hospital includes multiple levels of post-acute care in the meeting, the group becomes too large and has too many competing interests.

This clutter can make it more difficult to cover the business at hand. Some organizations have taken to having a post-acute care network meeting for SNFs and a separate meeting for home health, home care, hospice, palliative care, and assisted-living providers. This approach can also be effective. However, if your network includes a hospital-owned home health and hospice provider, it is much easier to have one post-acute care network meeting and include the hospital-based home health and hospice providers along with the SNFs.

Post-acute care network meetings should be invitation-only to make sure only the relevant stakeholders attend. These meetings are designed to give existing referral sources and post-acute care providers an opportunity to improve care coordination processes and tactics. Post-acute care providers that are not already receiving referrals or are not currently in the network should be required to generate referrals before they start regularly attending the meetings. These meetings are also not the correct forum for marketers who are trying to generate referrals and new business.

As a nursing home administrator, I worked in a community that held a quarterly post-acute care network meeting referred to as the "senior network." The location rotated through different SNFs but was hosted and coordinated by the local hospital. These meetings took place almost ten years before the ACA, so the goal then was to build a sense of community among the providers—a commendable approach that was well ahead of its time. Because the luncheons were held at SNFs and were open to all community providers who wanted to attend, however, the meetings were more a social function than a business event.

A few years later, when I became a hospital CEO, I replicated this program by creating a senior network in Anaheim, California. However, I made sure the new network luncheons were hosted at the hospital so that I could control who attended, and I tried to keep the invitation list to providers the hospital was already working with (to avoid the appearance of a social activity). Even before the ACA, these monthly, bimonthly, or quarterly meetings brought members of the care continuum together.

The meetings became a place to raise questions. I recall that at an Anaheim senior network meeting in 2006, an SNF administrator asked, "Why does your hospital send a higher volume of patients to long-term acute care (LTAC) hospitals after discharge than your competitors?" From my nursing home administrator days I knew how frustrating such a practice can be when you are trying to manage your census and bed availability. I explained that physicians have the ability to bill Medicare every day if they visit a patient in an LTAC hospital, whereas at an SNF their ability to collect reimbursement is limited to one day a week and then later just one day a month. I did not offer an opinion on whether this was the best care plan for the patients, but I could explain the fee-for-service reimbursement model and how many physicians used it to their financial advantage. This example illustrates that many times a problem has site-specific reasons. In this case, the administrator who asked the question did not realize that her own medical director, who had a strong relationship with a local LTAC hospital, was writing referrals to the LTAC hospital and fueling her frustration. I was able to share these details one-on-one rather than with the whole group. I share this story to give an example of how effective post-acute care network and community collaboratives have been even before the ACA in helping to exchange ideas and discuss ways to improve the care continuum.

NARROW THE HOSPITAL'S PROVIDER NETWORK

As a result of several of the initiatives in the ACA, health plans have once again become more aggressive in narrowing their provider network. What does that mean? Developing a narrow network means developing a list of preferred (or contracted) providers. Narrow networks have been evolving over several years, but the ACA has led more hospitals to narrow their post-acute care provider network. No magic formula exists for determining how many SNFs to include in your network, however. Each market and community will be different.

One of the main reasons acute care hospitals have begun narrowing their networks is to control their ability to coordinate care with post-acute care providers. By limiting the post-acute care providers in the post-acute care network, acute care hospitals are able to work directly with each provider on a weekly basis to manage quality and reduce unnecessary readmissions. If too many SNFs and home health agencies were in the mix, the hospital would not have the resources to meet and share as much data and information with each facility or agency every week.

How Do You Choose Network Members?

What key criteria should hospitals or health systems use in selecting network members? Though this question does not have a simple answer, there are two constants:

- A reputation for consistent quality
- A proven long-term track record in the community (longevity)

Proximity also plays a role, as do physician referral patterns. Each of these factors needs to be considered. Competitive pressures, such as other hospitals being closer to the facility than your hospital, should also be considered, as should contract penetration (aligning managed care contracts with the SNFs). Because hospitals and health systems want to negotiate a low rate of reimbursement with providers that have a long history of delivering successful results in the community, providers that have been in the community for several years have the advantage and are likely to become providers of choice.

Obviously, quality should be the number one factor and can never be compromised, but identifying which quality metrics and standards should be adhered to can be tricky because each provider will point to the metric it does best and suggest that the hospital use it as the benchmark. For example, a client that was narrowing its SNF network had a choice between a five-star SNF (according to CMS Hospital Compare) and a competing SNF with only a three-star rating but an effective disease-specific specialty program with documented success of reducing readmissions. The three-star facility (300 beds) claimed that it was not on a level playing field with the five-star facility (66 beds) because it took more complex patients as a result of its size.

I worked with a client that toured 13 SNFs in its area before narrowing its post-acute care network of SNFs to seven. The administrator of one of the facilities that was not included contacted the hospital to ask why his facility was not included. He cited his facility's quality initiatives and long history of partnering with the hospital. The hospital referred the administrator to me. The reasons I gave him are common factors in the decision to exclude an SNF from a network. First, not only was he closer to a competing hospital than he was to my client's hospital, but he was on the opposite side of the other hospital from my client's facility. This meant that county paramedic requirements would have to be breached to take a patient to my client's hospital if the patient needed acute care. Although that specific county honors patient choice, the paramedics are often required to take the patient to the nearest receiving hospital. Second, the per diem (paid by the insurance companies to the hospital) of the large neighboring hospital was significantly higher than that of any other hospital in the area, including my client's. Many health plans would therefore try to keep their patients away from SNFs in the 911 zone of that specific hospital. I encouraged him to contact the neighboring hospital to suggest that they start a post-acute care network.

Although this conversation was not an easy one, it exemplifies what is to come in the post-acute care sector over the next few years.

In short, not only does the ACA incentivize us to coordinate care with post-acute care providers, but it also becomes a market-share play when you willingly send your patients into your competitor's primary service area and expose them to physicians, health plans, and other providers that are all anxious to prove they can care for the patient better than you can. For all of those reasons, coordinating care and narrowing your network of post-acute care providers is important.

Unfortunately, providers that are not included in narrow networks are likely to see a decline in volume and referrals over the next few years. Many will have difficulty staying in business, especially in states that are working to phase out the fee-for-service model by converting dually covered patients into managed care. Many states have fast-tracked initiatives to get themselves out of the insurance business as soon as possible. Recent history has shown that forcing everyone who has historically been in the fee-for-service program into managed care results in savings for the payer and less overhead for the state and federal government. These programs are commonly referred to as "dual" programs because the beneficiaries are dually eligible for both Medicare and Medicaid.

Narrow the Network of Home Health Agencies

Narrowing your network of home health agencies is as important as narrowing your SNF network. In fact, narrowing your network of home health agencies may be even more critical because the trend is to care for patients at home who were previously cared for at an acute care hospital. Working with more than three home health agencies is a significant burden for a health plan or hospital. More important, coordinating care with multiple providers will eventually become an unnecessary burden. Although historically many hospitals owned and operated a home health agency, many were shut down in the 1990s and 2000s as home health proved to be a low-margin, high-risk service line. Many hospitals are now turning back to operating their own home health agency because it is a more efficient means of managing patients in a coordinated care model.

Coordinating care with even one home health agency can be time consuming and difficult. Even several years after the strictly fee-for-service model, operators continue to struggle to identify how to consistently coordinate care between providers. To simplify: The fewer providers there are, the simpler it becomes to coordinate care. As long as the home health providers are exceeding identified quality benchmarks, you will likely continue to see a trend toward system-based home health agencies.

ALIGN CONTRACTS WITH POST-ACUTE CARE NETWORK MEMBERS

Post-acute care providers must ensure that they have the same managed care (health plan) contracts as their acute hospital referral sources. This is even more important in states where traditional Medicare fee-for-service patients are being pushed into managed care organizations' dual programs. The fee-for-service model of the past will likely go away permanently in states such as California and New York. Many post-acute care providers have only cared for fee-for-service patients and have not had to deal with such situations as getting a preauthorization before providing care to a patient, but the change to a managed care model is likely to be fully implemented in some states as early as 2017. Providers should make sure they are prepared to succeed in an environment where fee-for-service patients no longer exist and they are required to get a preauthorization on every patient before they can provide care.

The new model also means lower reimbursement for post-acute care providers in the coming years because managed care providers will seek the lowest bidder when selecting post-acute care partners for their narrow network. Yet the health plan and managed care partners will still require that the provider have a proven track record of delivering quality care.

All post-acute providers should view the federal government's push toward enrolling all fee-for-service patients in managed care as a significant threat. It ultimately leads to lower reimbursement than they received in the days of the fee-for-service model and shorter lengths of stay. In addition, post-acute care providers will see their administrative costs rise as preauthorizations and additional paperwork become the norm, even with the benefit of electronic health records. Further, more staff time will be required to obtain the authorizations and extensions caretakers need to effectively and safely discharge patients home after a post-acute care episode.

The most important takeaway from this section is this: If your post-acute care organization is not already moving to contract with the hospital or payer in your community as part of a narrow network, it may already be too late. This is especially true of SNFs and home health agencies. For the sake of the long-term well-being of your post-acute care organization, align yourself with all payers in your market and work vigilantly until you have done so.

Payers, hospitals, health systems, health plans, and managed-care organizations will make this issue a priority. Once a health plan already has two or three contracted providers in a certain market, it may not see a need to add more facilities. Another contract just becomes additional, unnecessary work. This is also true for home health and hospice agencies. Your quality, your success at reducing readmissions, and your effective disease-specific programs are in large part all irrelevant to the health plan if it already has enough capacity to handle its patient population in your market area, because value-added quality programs have come to be expected of contract partners. Only rarely are specialty programs enough to convince a health plan to add another post-acute care provider if it thinks it already has enough capacity in a market. Adding another post-acute care provider simply because it stands above its peers is rarely a priority for a health system, health plan, or managed care organization that already has enough capacity at that post-acute care level.

IMPLEMENT A TRANSITIONAL CARE PROGRAM

In addition to narrow networks, many hospitals have also implemented a transitional care program. Transitional care programs are at the heart of the intent of the ACA and are one of the six programs that incentivize hospitals to coordinate care. Many hospitals are using transitional care programs to narrow their networks to include only preferred providers. Although transitional care programs accomplish essentially the same goal as post-acute care networks, they are a more formal means of narrowing the network and make a strong statement that the hospital is committed to partnering with select post-acute care providers.

A transitional care program aligns the interests of the post-acute care providers with those of the hospital, health system, and health plan. In addition to the preferred providers in the narrow network, a transitional care program includes an ambulatory case manager (often called a "navigator" or a "coach" in the Coleman Care Transitions model) to follow each patient and manage her care at each destination, including once she is back home or in an assisted-living environment. The distinct advantages of transitional care programs are enhanced communication among physicians, nurses, therapists, and case managers; between levels of care; and with the ambulatory case manager (navigator) who is assigned to monitor the patient after discharge from the hospital. Although acute and post-acute care providers are still finding their way in terms of enhancing their ability to communicate about an individual patient's care, great strides are being made, and all levels of care are being incentivized in a value-based reimbursement model.

Transitional care programs are another reason hospitals and health systems are looking to narrow their network of post-acute care providers. When a hospital offers a patient the opportunity to enter a transitional care program at no additional cost, there must be a value proposition illustrating the enhanced level of care the patient receives by entering the transitional care program. That value proposition includes not only enhanced communication but also a higher level of care through partnering with post-acute care providers in the narrow network. Other benefits include a single electronic platform (health information exchange), data sharing, the ability to continue with a patient's physician of choice (to the extent possible), and, in the near future, the availability of a patient's data in an electronic health record should that patient ever return to the emergency department.

One example of a successful venture in coordinating care is Sharp Healthcare, which partnered with Shea Family Homes, a chain of SNFs in the San Diego area, under the brand Sharp Extended Care. Even though the nursing homes are owned by Shea Family Homes and remain independent, the two organizations partnered to create a transitional care program that appears to the patients as a well-managed coordinated care program. Hospitals are beginning to realize that they can honor patient choice and anti-steering regulations and at the same time narrow their post-acute care networks through an effective transitional care program.

Several hospitals have gone so far as to embed a prepopulated order in the physician notes area of a patient's chart allowing the doctor to order "care transitions" as an option instead of just writing "discharge to a skilled-nursing facility." The care transitions option allows navigators to go to the bedside and share with the patient the details of the care transitions program. Although federal antisteering regulations require case managers to give patients a complete list of post-acute care providers, a quality transitional care program brochure is one way to narrow the network. If the hospital provides patients with the full list of post-acute care providers along with this brochure using a well-prepared script, the patients will almost always choose the transitional care program and the hospital will have complied with federal choice and antisteering regulations.

Narrowing networks and implementing transitional care programs are a significant threat to many post-acute care providers that have thrived under a fee-for-service model. However, the growth of home health providers is likely to plateau and lead to a significant decline in agencies over the next few years. Home health agencies will find it difficult to survive if they are not in a narrow network because hospitals and health systems will likely narrow their coordinated care networks to a single system-owned agency or a small network of three to five home health agencies.

When I speak at national healthcare events, I share my belief that we will see a significant thinning of home health providers in the near future. My message is simple: If you are not embedded with a health system or payer now, you are at great risk of losing volume to the point of extinction over the next few years. Many home health providers in the audience are disappointed by this message, and for this reason several of my colleagues jokingly refer to me as the "doomsday speaker" on the readmissions circuit. That makes me laugh, but I understand their point. Not many people are willing to say it as clearly and firmly as I do, but because I have been on all sides of the continuum of care (as a nursing home and assisted-living administrator, hospital CEO, and acute rehab CEO) and over both home health and hospice, I have a unique perspective on what the future model will bring.

PROMOTE PATIENT CHOICE AND ADHERE TO ANTISTEERING REGULATIONS

At a speaking engagement in 2013, I stated that hospitals that have a well-written transitional care brochure and accompanying consent form for patients to sign are in fact "champions for patient choice." After the presentation, someone asked me, "What do you believe qualifies an organization as a champion for patient choice?" My response? Organizations that develop a brochure that lists their preferred providers (narrow network) and educates patients about their choices are acting as champions for choice because few hospitals have patients sign anything confirming their choice of post-acute care providers. The consent form allows patients to confirm in writing that they were aware they had a choice of post-acute care providers. The consent form also confirms that the patient was given a complete list of providers and allows the patient to consent to those choices in writing.

Hospitals are using transitional care programs as a means to keep patients in a coordinated care model. However, regulations requiring hospitals to honor a patient's choice when selecting a post-acute care provider and federal antisteering regulations are still in place. In fact, all providers (e.g., hospital, SNF, home health) that become Medicare participants agree to adhere to these regulations as a condition of participation in the Medicare reimbursement program. These regulations contradict the intent of the ACA—which is to coordinate care and to reimburse for care based on value, not episode (as was prevalent under the fee-for-service model). Perhaps the biggest dilemma in coordinating care in a post-ACA environment is how to coordinate care without steering.

To address this dilemma, let's start by discussing the intent of the patient choice and antisteering regulations. The regulations were created to prevent and discourage unfair business practices, to create transparency, and to ensure patient choice. Patients had to be informed of whether a physician had a financial interest in an SNF, home health agency, or board-and-care facility, but the attempt to ensure transparency was not limited to physicians—many post-acute care providers would place relatives and spouses in jobs at hospitals, medical groups, and health plans with high-volume discharges to steer patients to their agency. Anyone who has worked in case management, discharge planning, or the post-acute care sector has encountered conflicts of interest of this nature.

At one point I was considering asking CMS for a legal opinion on the topic of antisteering, but a healthcare attorney I was consulting with said, "What if they tell you what you don't want to hear?" As I thought about his response, I came to the conclusion that there must be a way to design a program that honors patient choice, does not steer, and meets both the letter and the spirit of the law of the choice and antisteering regulations. Later I met an attorney who had actually asked representatives from CMS how care could be coordinated without steering. Their response? He said they were unwilling to answer it. I chuckled and said, "Of course. We knew the answer before you even asked."

Although the Medicare Payment Advisory Commission (MedPAC 2014) has discussed the steering regulations as being antiquated and in need of change, hospitals must continue to identify creative ways to coordinate care and at the same time honor these outdated regulations. For example, a number of health systems in Florida tightened their security measures and do not allow post-acute care providers on campus at all.

The most important step any hospital or health system can take to address the choice and antisteering issue when designing a transitions program is to involve the compliance officer and healthcare attorneys in the process. Trying to find a way to narrow the network and not violate patient choice and antisteering regulations is one of the most common frustrations among providers at present and one of the most frequent questions I get when speaking at national events. The best answer I can offer is to adhere to the antisteering regulations by getting patients' consent and an acknowledgment that the patients were offered a complete list of providers, had a choice, and selected the identified facilities and agencies.

FORM COMMUNITY COALITIONS

Another common tactic being implemented in healthcare organizations is the formation of community coalitions of hospitals and post-acute care providers. The purpose of such coalitions is to improve care coordination, but in contrast to the post-acute network model, in which one hospital is in the driver's seat, community coalitions involve multiple hospitals. In addition, their efforts are often focused on standardizing practices and implementing best-practice protocols to coordinate care and prevent readmissions. Often, Medicare-mandated state quality improvement organizations will help facilitate these coalitions in the community.

In the initial planning stages of a community coalition, I advise starting with a small group of key influencers, including

- the high-volume hospital,
- the SNFs the hospitals use most frequently, and
- one to three of the highest-volume home health agencies.

If you keep the initial planning group to fewer than 30 people, identify objectives and tactics for the coalition, and then invite other community providers, the coalition is much more likely to achieve sustainable growth and results.

Once the community coalition is past the planning stage and ready to expand, be sure to include all of the hospitals in the community—both large and small. The larger hospitals refer the highest volume of patients to post-acute care and will ultimately drive the success of the coalition because post-acute care providers pay the most attention to them. On the other hand, though they have less clout with post-acute care providers, smaller hospitals are often more willing to champion the coalition's efforts. Other entities that should be included are the private health plans, contract partners, managed care organizations, and post-acute care providers in the community. Providers ranging from SNFs to LTAC hospitals, acute rehab, home health, hospice, home care, palliative care, and even assisted-living facilities should be welcomed and invited to participate in the coalition. Although all community coalitions need engaged members to drive the mission and initiatives, community coalitions in large urban areas often face additional challenges of geographic variation and extreme distances between providers.

Once multiple hospitals and post-acute care providers are at the table, it can be difficult to manage competing initiatives and get them to agree on a single set of goals and tactics for the coalition.

But when you have successfully attracted both acute and post-acute providers to the coalition, it has a much greater chance of success.

Ultimately, it is the health plan or payer that benefits financially from the improved care continuum as patient transfers become more fluid as a result of the improved communication between facilities and as patients' lengths of stay shorten, allowing them to return home sooner. Although the patient benefits from the improved quality, without the input and support of the organization—that is, the party that is hit the hardest financially—it is more difficult to create a sustainable model that will provide consistent results. This is a simple supply-and-demand proposition. Post-acute care facilities and agencies rely on the high-volume acute care hospital for the volume that will sustain their business model. If they do not embrace the goals and objectives of the high-volume referral source, post-acute care providers will see a decline in volume to the point that they can no longer operate.

DEVELOP A SECONDARY-MARKET POST-ACUTE CARE PROVIDER LIST

Developing a secondary-market post-acute care provider list is an interesting but seldom implemented tactic that hospitals should consider. In one hospital I was working with, I noticed that of its five readmissions in one month, three came from one SNF that was not in its narrow network and only two came from one of the eight SNFs in its established post-acute care network. I realized that hospitals are at greater risk for readmissions from SNFs that are not in their narrow network. So how do you address this problem? First, you find out why a physician referred a patient to a facility outside the narrow network to begin with. That should happen only sparingly.

One way to address the problem of out-of-network SNFs not implementing tactics to avoid readmissions is to develop a secondary-market post-acute care provider list. In addition to its list of providers in the immediate market, a hospital should consider identifying high-quality skilled-nursing partners in outlying areas in case a patient asks to go to a nursing home closer to his residence. For example, Orange County, California, is a 50- to 60-minute commute to downtown Los Angeles, where many Orange County residents work. If an employee has an accident or is hospitalized during the day and then needs post-acute care, the patient is more likely to choose a facility in an outlying area. Therefore, identifying a handful of facilities in outlying areas that have implemented software and protocols for reporting and predicting readmissions is a tactic many hospitals should consider.

ENCOURAGE PATIENT SELF-MANAGEMENT

Most thought leaders in the coordinated-care space would agree that the most important factor in eliminating readmissions is a patient's ability to care for herself. If patients understand their options and are able to take better care of themselves at home, readmission penalties will likely never come about because readmissions would not be a problem. Many of the technologies and solutions being introduced to the industry focus on helping patients better care for themselves in a home environment.

Research suggests that social issues such as anxiety, access to transportation, self-isolation, depression, dehydration, and improper nutrition are the leading reasons patients are readmitted to hospitals unnecessarily (Kilroy, Morgan-Solomon, and Landrum 2013). If patients understand their personal challenges and educate themselves on how to self-manage, the issue of unnecessary readmissions would be significantly reduced. This book does not focus on this issue at length because self-management is more of a coordinated-care initiative, but executives should be aware of the issue when identifying readmission prevention solutions.

PROMOTE PATIENT HEALTH LITERACY AND USE TEACH-BACK METHODS

Promoting patient health literacy is another major tactic in effectively coordinating care. A patient must understand his challenges, barriers, and needs before he can effectively self-manage his care. All providers and caretakers across the continuum are responsible for educating patients. This often presents additional challenges because the fee-for-service model created an environment of independence and lack of communication between providers. As a result, patients—even those who wanted to better understand their personal needs and how to best care for themselves—often got conflicting messages from doctors, pharmacists, therapists, and caretakers. These providers had no financial incentive to communicate.

One of the most common tactics hospitals are implementing to combat the readmission issue is "teach-back." Teach-back is effective in educating patients how to self-manage their care after they leave the hospital and is a means of making sure the patient understands the steps she needs to take to care for herself once she returns home. The procedure is for an educator to ask the patient to recite the information related to her care to confirm that she has a clear understanding of the discharge plan and prescribed medication regimen. Readmission and population management problems could be solved if patients learned to care for themselves properly. Haney and Shepherd (2013) showed that teach-back can be effective in reducing a hospital's readmission rate. Patient self-management can be the most effective tactic if a patient and his caregiver comprehend the plan of care.

Teach-back can be difficult because social issues, including shyness, anxiety, language barriers, educational impediments, and physical impairments (such as seniors who speak softly), can be an impediment. Although many hospitals have social workers, navigators, liaisons, or coaches in addition to case managers, and all of them use this tactic—particularly with high-risk patients—patient engagement remains one of the top challenges to providing efficient coordinated care and preventing unnecessary readmissions.

COLLECT FACILITY-SPECIFIC DATA

In the war on unnecessary readmissions, you can never have enough data. Initially, readmissions data specific to your facility may seem hard to come by, but facility-specific data are not as scarce as you might think. Between your state's CMS-mandated quality improvement organization (see Chapter 2) and your state's hospital and nursing home trade association, enough facility-specific data are available to identify problem areas. One of the biggest challenges is the delay in securing timely data from the federal database. Typically, there is a 12-month delay for facility-specific data unless the hospital has implemented RightCare Solutions software or another software package that provides real-time data.

That said, collecting your own data is also critical. The hospital can likely pull a significant amount of its own readmission data from its software and electronic health record. Although some facilities have found that their systems are not set up to collect readmission data, many others have found that the collection process can be entirely automated. Although data extracted from the electronic health record is specific to same-hospital readmission rates, hospitals can use their same-hospital return rate ratio as an indicator of overall readmission volume to project an estimated rate. These data are available in the hospital's annual report from CMS.

For example, say Hospital A has a 79.9 percent same-hospital return rate in January 2015 and Hospital A's monthly internal readmissions log for January shows 40 readmissions. If 40 same-hospital readmissions represents 79.9 percent of the facility's overall readmissions, then Hospital A's expected overall readmissions for January would be approximately 50. One of the major challenges here is that the actual readmission rate for January from the claims database may take an additional 12 months to secure. Again, this is why developing a facility-specific data collection plan is important.

Hospitals and health systems should also ask partner SNFs to track readmission information, share it regularly at meetings, and then compile a monthly report for the hospital. If the hospital is not consistently asking post-acute care providers to track and submit these data on a monthly basis, the data are not likely to be collected consistently. SNFs that are focused on quality, communication, coordinated care, and readmission prevention should be able to track all readmissions with relative ease. If they are tracking and logging all patients who return to the emergency department, then those who end up being readmitted should be easily identified, and there should be, at most, a few each month.

Other post-acute care providers, including home health and hospice agencies, LTAC hospitals, inpatient rehabilitation facilities, and assisted-living facilities, should all track their own readmissions and share the information with the acute care provider. These comprehensive data will help providers better identify trends, referral patterns, and risk factors. Post-acute care providers that are not tracking and sharing readmission data with acute care referral partners are now in the minority. Further, a lack of commitment to data collection is a sure sign that a post-acute care facility is falling short on the hospital's quality expectations. Acute and post-acute care providers should all be collecting, sharing, and discussing internal readmissions data monthly even though the sources and specific data being researched may differ slightly. Without a consistent commitment to using specific data, it will be difficult to identify focus areas and emerging trends for the group to collaborate on in improving the coordinated care model.

Several mainstream software companies generate automated reports for SNFs. American HealthTech, Servarus, PointRight, and COMS Interactive are software products whose reports have been successfully used and marketed by SNFs to acute care partners (see Exhibit 3.1 for a sample report). Though other products

Exhibit 3.1 Sample Readmission Report

St. Lucas
Healthcare Community

Clinical Update – September 2014

Use Health Information to Proactively Drive Care and Improve Performance

Becoming a market leader in improving clinical outcomes and cost-effectiveness requires integrated health care networks to optimize performance through systematic and comprehensive use of health-related knowledge. This is particularly true when managing chronic disease and assuming the associated risk in a bundled payment environment.

One strategy for improving outcomes, quality, value, and satisfaction is to implement clinical decision support (CDS) technology. CDS technology delivers necessary information in a timely manner, usually at the point of care, to inform decisions about a patient's care. Examples of CDS capabilities include:

- A guided clinical assessment, tailored to each patient's disease and risk profiles.
- Care recommendations and care plans developed with the assistance of a clinical rules engine.
- Embedded evidence-based guidelines and order sets reducing variations in patterns of clinical care.
- Consistency in data collection that enables effective and efficient quality improvement initiatives.
- Connecting the care team with decision support tools.

Clinical Technology Helped our Center Achieve Great Clinical Outcomes

St. Lucas Healthcare's excellent clinical outcomes are a direct result of our advanced disease management program, which leverages Daylight IQ™ to provide the post-acute population with a higher quality of care. The following chart illustrates lower return to hospital and mortality rates St. Lucas Healthcare is achieving, as compared to county, state and national averages.

Resident Discharge Profile	St. Lucas Healthcare Average[1]	Rice County Average[3]	Minnesota State Average[2]	U.S. National Average
< 30 Day Return to Hospital	7.7%	21.0%	19.1%	23.5%[3]
< 30 Day Mortality Rate	2.2%	10.3%	11.8%	12.6%[2]

[1] Reflects clinical data 8/1/13 - 8/1/14.

[2] Source: Medicare.gov, Hospital Outcome of Care Measures.

[3] Source: *Revolving Door of Rehospitalization from Skilled Nursing Facilities*, Mor, Intrator, et al, Health Affairs, Jan 2010.

St. Lucas Healthcare Community's Areas of Clinical Focus

The St. Lucas Healthcare clinical staff is addressing complex disease profiles, and providing an advanced clinical focus in the following areas:

• General	• Ortho/Musculoskeletal	• Cardiovascular
• Infectious	• Pulmonary	• Neurologic

Care Reminder – Aspiration Pneumonia

Two basic interventions, both cornerstones of nursing practice, are key to reducing the risk of aspiration pneumonia: 1) maintaining head of bed at 30° or greater and 2) adhering to a systematic oral health care schedule. For more information about aspiration pneumonia and additional prevention strategies, please visit http://www.nlm.nih.gov/medlineplus/aspirationpneumonia.

St. Lucas Healthcare Community ♦ 500 SE 1st Street, Rice, Minnesota 55021 ♦ Tel: (507) 332-5100

(continued)

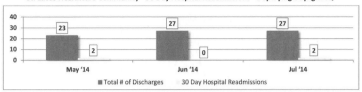

COMS Interactive™ Clinical Update – September 2014 Edition

St. Lucas Healthcare Community - 30 Day Hospital Readmissions - Deploying Daylight IQ™

Chart data: May '14: 23 Total # of Discharges, 2 30 Day Hospital Readmissions; Jun '14: 27, 0; Jul '14: 27, 2

■ Total # of Discharges ▪ 30 Day Hospital Readmissions

St. Lucas Healthcare Community - Outcomes Measurements by Disease Category

Disease Category Profile	Total	Home	Assisted Living	Long Term Care	Hospital Readmit <30 days	Hospital Readmit >30 days	Expired <30 Days	Expired >30 Days	Other[1]
Cancer	0	-	-	-	-	-	-	-	-
Cardiovascular	6	4	-	1	-	1	-	-	-
Eye, Ear, Nose, Throat	0	-	-	-	-	-	-	-	-
Gastrointestinal	1	1	-	-	-	-	-	-	-
General	230	105	22	47	20	4	6	2	24
Genitourinary	0	-	-	-	-	-	-	-	-
Immune	0	-	-	-	-	-	-	-	-
Infectious	5	1	-	2	-	1	-	-	1
Metabolic/Endocrine	0	-	-	-	-	-	-	-	-
Neurologic	4	1	-	2	-	-	-	-	1
Ortho/Musculoskeletal	16	9	2	2	1	-	-	-	2
Psychiatric	1	1	-	-	-	-	-	-	-
Pulmonary	4	2	-	2	-	-	-	-	-
Renal	0	-	-	-	-	-	-	-	-
Skin	3	2	1	-	-	-	-	-	-
Other	1	1	-	-	-	-	-	-	-
Total Skilled Discharges	**271**	**127**	**25**	**56**	**21**	**6**	**6**	**2**	**28**
Reflects clinical data 8/1/13 - 8/1/14. [1] Other includes: LTAC, AMA, hospice and planned hospital procedures.		46.9%	9.2%	20.7%	7.7%	2.2%	2.2%	0.7%	10.3%

St. Lucas Healthcare Community - Outcomes Measurements vs. Region - Medicare Areas of Focus

Readmission and Mortality	St. Lucas Healthcare Average[1]	Rice County Average[2]	Minnesota State Average[2]	U. S. National Average[2]
Heart Attack	0/0 = 0.0%	Data Not Available	34.4%	35.7%
Heart Failure	0/1 = 0.0%	32.5%	36.1%	36.1%
Pneumonia	0/3 = 0.0%	27.4%	30.0%	30.3%
COPD	0/0 = 0.0%	Identified as the next clinically-focused diagnosis.		
Hip & Knee Replacement	0/3 = 0.0%	CMS has defined as a key diagnosis.		

[1] Reflects clinical data 8/1/13 - 8/1/14.
[2] Source: Medicare.gov, Hospital Outcome of Care Measures.

This report is intended for informational purposes only. Industry standard data analysis processes and methodologies have been used to validate and present the information. The process for compiling information from user source documents and/or source data is compliant with The Health Insurance Portability and Accountability Act of 1996 (HIPAA). This report is not meant to be absolute and may be updated and/or modified as appropriate.

St. Lucas Healthcare Community ♦ 500 SE 1st Street, Rice, Minnesota 55021 ♦ Tel: (507) 332-5100

Source: COMS Interactive and Welcov Healthcare. Used with permission.

can provide summaries and reports, those named here are specific to readmission prevention, and SNFs are using them to generate monthly readmission reports to share with hospital partners. Of all the marketing tactics SNFs can use to set themselves apart from their competition, monthly delivery of these reports to hospital referral partners may be the most beneficial.

REFERENCES

Bowles, K. 2014. Personal communication with the author, May 7.

Haney, M., and J. Shepherd. 2013. "Can Teach-Back Reduce Hospital Readmissions?" *American Nurse Today* 9 (3): 50–52.

Kilroy, C., D. Morgan-Solomon, and P. Landrum. 2013. Accessed December 15, 2014. *Preventing Patient Rebounds.* Optum Health white paper. www.optum.com/content/dam /optum/resources/whitePapers/ReadmissionPrevention _WhitePaper_Online_FINAL.pdf.

Medicare Payment Advisory Commission (MedPAC). 2014. "Public Meeting." Transcript of meeting held October 9, 2014, Washington, DC. www.medpac.gov/documents /october-2014-meeting-transcript.pdf.

CHAPTER 4

Prevention Planning Phase Two: After Discharge

The second phase of planning to prevent unnecessary readmissions focuses on postdischarge tactics—what happens after the patient leaves the hospital. Just as in Phase One, Phase Two offers operators of healthcare facilities at all levels a chance to collaborate. Acute care providers should join with nursing homes, home health providers, hospice and palliative care providers, assisted-living facilities, and other community resources to help patients better manage their own care. Many of the tactics discussed here can be employed in the absence of the post-acute care networks described as a tactic in Phase One. However, if your hospital has or is considering forming a post-acute care network, discuss with your team how your network can incorporate the tactics described here.

PERFORM A MEDICATION RECONCILIATION

Because, in many modern hospitals, a comprehensive health information exchange to provide real-time personalized patient data is often lacking and hospitalist models remain prevalent, patients often do not know the physician treating them in the hospital and a new regimen of medications is prescribed. As a result, patients and their family members may be confused about which regimen to follow after returning home. Thus, medication reconciliation is one of the most significant challenges that leads to unnecessary hospitalization and readmissions.

Many programs and technologies have emerged to help with medication reconciliation. For example, Einstein Medical Center in Philadelphia developed the Medication REACH (Reconciliation, Education, Access, Counseling, Healthy Patient at Home) program when it made a calculated decision to focus on medication adherence and compliance as a key driver of avoidable readmissions. The result was a readmission rate that dropped from 21.4 percent in the control group to 10.6 percent in the REACH group (see the Medication REACH case example in Appendix B for a complete summary).

Medication reconciliation is a major component of the transitional care programs discussed later in this book, and hospitals and health systems have taken many approaches to address this problem. Companies such as Walgreens and CVS have created service lines to work with hospitals to better address the medication reconciliation problem. CheckMeds is another company that has implemented national models to collaborate with hospitals to better manage medication reconciliation. Medication reconciliation can also be done at the patient's postdischarge follow-up visit with her physician.

SCHEDULE POST-ACUTE CARE FOLLOW-UP VISITS

Preparing hospital patients to self-manage their care when they return home is essential. Patients are most vulnerable immediately after discharge from the hospital and are likely to experience increased pain, confusion, anxiety, and depression (Tam et al. 2014). Of the many models for conducting post-acute care visits, the most prevalent are (1) a primary care physician office visit, (2) a post-acute care clinic visit, or (3) a home visit. Each of those three models will be discussed later in this section.

The two main goals of the post-acute care visit are to (1) get an update on the patient's well-being (after returning to her normal living environment or a lower level of care) and (2) do an exhaustive reconciliation of all prescribed medications. Once the physician (or, in some cases, a pharmacist, physician assistant, or nurse practitioner) has reviewed and reconciled all of the patient's medications, the new regimen should be discussed with the patient and/or family member. Often, teach-back methods are used to confirm that the patient understands the purpose and usage of each medication. The reconciliation is also an opportunity to discuss medication side effects and potential harmful interactions with other prescribed medications.

Primary Care Physician Office Visit

At the follow-up visit, the primary care physician should ask a series of questions to ensure that the patient was safely transitioned home and is not experiencing any unforeseen challenges. After a brief discussion to address those concerns, the remainder of the appointment is spent doing a medication reconciliation and developing a new daily drug regimen for the patient. Patients should be asked to bring all medications in their possession to the appointment, with the goal being for them to leave with a clear direction and understanding of their new medication plan.

Most important, the physician's goal is to address any anxiety the patient is having about his personal care plan and to provide him with instructions, support, resources, and supplies so he can best care for himself at home. Because the patient and physician often have a long-standing relationship, this model can be effective if the primary care physician understands the goal of the post-acute care visit.

The biggest challenge in implementing a model relying on primary care physicians is educating physicians about the unique characteristics of a post-acute care visit and equipping them with the appropriate materials. Although Medicare reimburses physicians for conducting post-acute care visits, many physicians conduct them so seldom that health systems find it difficult to effectively implement this model. Systems that have been able to get primary care physicians on board, however, have found this model to be one of the most effective tools in reducing readmissions.

Post-Acute Care Clinic Visit

A number of hospitals and health systems use a post-acute care clinic, also called a care coordination clinic, for patient follow-up. This type of visit is preferable when poor communication exists between the hospitalist and primary care physician (who may not even know the patient was hospitalized). Thus, all Medicare patients who are discharged from the hospital, emergency department (ED), or local skilled-nursing facility (SNF) are encouraged to go to the post-acute care clinic for a follow-up visit.

After the patient's visit to the clinic, the physician, pharmacist, nurse practitioner, or physician assistant completes a postdischarge visit summary, which is forwarded to the patient's primary care physician. Eventually, when electronic health records are fully implemented, this summary will also be input into the record and available to the hospital, primary care physician, coordinated care clinic, hospital-owned home health and hospice agencies, and local nursing homes (should the patient ever be admitted to an SNF). The clinic physician should also place a courtesy call to the primary care physician after the visit to update her on the patient's status.

In the future, post-acute care clinics will likely become high-risk clinics for the most part. These high-risk clinics would not only fulfill the role of the post-acute care clinic but also evolve into the patient-centered medical home for all the patient's primary care and medication reconciliation needs.

Home Visit

Many health plans and medical groups send a physician or a physician extender (a mid-level practitioner, such as a physician assistant or nurse practitioner) into the home to conduct the post-acute care visit. The intent of the home visit is the same as the office visit. However, in the home there is a greater opportunity to identify risk factors, such as pets, staircases, and items that could be tripping hazards. The clinician is also able to identify signs of self-isolation, hoarding, malnourishment, and other issues that may affect the patient's care plan.

The home visit model is likely to become more prevalent as organizations identify more cost-efficient means of visiting patients in the home—particularly high-risk patients. Several emerging models for home visits integrate an entire network of ancillary providers. In one emerging model, the SNF group extends its services into the home to shorten the SNF length of stay and uses mid-level practitioners (nurse practitioners and physician assistants) who are already providing services at the SNF level. The biggest challenge facing home-based care models is the expense.

Traditionally, the community has turned to the local hospital to assume the risk of programs of this nature. However, with the diminishing inpatient census nationwide and accompanying diminishing revenues, hospital executives are looking to the health plans that now assume most of the risk for patient care to take on this responsibility. Though health plans are taking on this challenge, it is happening at a snail's pace.

In larger markets such as New York and Los Angeles, companies such as Medicast have started offering physician house calls via a mobile application on smart phones. Patients are guaranteed a home visit by a physician within three hours. Most of these visits are reimbursed privately by the patient, who enters a credit card number via the app. Insurers, Medicare, and Medicaid will likely seek to partner with similar organizations if the house-call model proves to be more effective and less costly than other alternatives.

SET UP HOME DELIVERY OF MEDICATIONS

Medication delivery programs have also proven beneficial in helping patients self-manage their care. Although patients have used mail-order medication delivery for years, some health systems have found it difficult to manage high-risk patients ordering medications through the mail. Others, however, have developed software or specialized programs to help patients with medication adherence. The programs send out reminders through such means as automated phone calls, live phone calls, e-mails, or text messages.

Recently, Walgreens and other local and national pharmacies have enhanced their home-delivery models at the request of health plans. This is another means of getting "eyes and ears" into a patient's home on a regular basis. Health plans are also developing new programs to get eyes and ears into their high-risk patients' homes as often as possible.

ESTABLISH AN AMBULATORY CASE MANAGEMENT SYSTEM

The term *ambulatory case management* refers to a system in which an ambulatory case manager (ACM) is assigned to a patient once he is discharged from the hospital. Just as managed care organizations have done for years, hospitals and ambulatory care organizations are now going to great lengths to monitor the well-being of their high-risk and other patients. The ACM monitors patients electronically and regularly visits and communicates with patients and caretakers. As electronic health records become more advanced, this task will become much easier as multiple caretakers can share data in real time and have access to a more comprehensive patient history. However, for most hospitals and ambulatory care organizations, the task of ambulatory case management remains laborious.

ACMs are assigned to patients while they are hospitalized and often participate in daily morning patient clinical rounds with nursing staff at the acute care hospital to best understand the patients' situation before discharge. The ACM also participates in rounds in post-acute care facilities, including SNFs, long-term acute care hospitals, and inpatient rehabilitation facilities, and communicates with each of the home health agencies providing care to high-risk patients. Each organization has a different set of timelines and expectations for its ACMs, but the underlying goal is the same: Communicate regularly with the patient and caretakers to ensure the patient has the knowledge and resources to remain in good health and avoid unnecessary rehospitalizations. The ACM has one of the most important roles in preventing unnecessary readmissions. If the ACM can effectively manage the patient outside of the hospital, the hospital is likely to see a significant reduction in readmissions.

The ACM often spends more time with the patient than the physician and thus may be able to suggest to a physician or caretaker an alternative approach that is more suitable for the patient than the standard course of action. For example, earlier I mentioned a patient who was readmitted to Johns Hopkins Medical more than 20 times in one year. The patient's ACM suggested that the physician provide the patient with a remote cardiac monitoring device. The intervention proved effective and was an option the physician had not considered until the ACM suggested it.

PROVIDE REMOTE MONITORING FOR THE PATIENT

Although telehealth and remote monitoring have been mainstream applications in Europe for many years, they remain uncharted territory for many US health systems. Many healthcare professionals think telehealth is a technology for rural areas or island communities with little access to physicians, but remote monitoring devices have also proven effective in preventing readmissions in urban areas, and most states have started reimbursing for telehealth.

Remote monitoring devices use Bluetooth or other technologies to communicate via a centralized command center. The communication can go directly to a hospital floor or, in some cases, to a call center (managed by a third party) that monitors communications for multiple health systems around the country. Most remote monitoring companies design readmission prevention programs for individual health systems to meet each health system's unique needs.

For example, remote monitoring can be used for patients with congestive heart failure. These patients are subject to rapid weight gain and loss, which is an early indicator of clinical symptoms. Patients would weigh themselves at home each morning on a scale equipped with Bluetooth technology that wirelessly reports the daily weight to a local operator.

POST-ACUTE CARE NETWORK TACTICS

After following the Phase One tactic of establishing a post-acute care network of facilities and providers, a number of tactics can be implemented for network members to meet a hospital's specific needs.

Schedule Regular Provider Meetings

Many hospitals host a monthly or bimonthly business meeting for post-acute care providers. Typically the meeting is a luncheon, but any format is acceptable. To keep the focus on business, it is important that the hospital or health system, and not an SNF, host the meeting so that the function does not turn into a marketing event or open house for an SNF. Post-acute care network meetings should be brief, have a concise agenda, and provide an update to each attendee regarding the group's success in coordinating care and preventing readmissions.

One method of assessing a member's success is to formally examine monthly or quarterly readmission rates for each facility. Although up-to-date readmission data may be difficult to obtain, it is still appropriate to share community readmission trends as much as a year later so that root-cause analyses can be performed. The hospital may also want to use the meeting as an opportunity to identify a focus area for the SNFs for each quarter. If, for example, data from the first quarter show a slight increase in readmissions for patients undergoing total knee and hip replacement, then these procedures would be the priority for network members for the next three months. Further, because SNFs often do not have the resources and educational materials that a hospital and health system may have access to, the meetings are an opportunity for continuing education.

In the foregoing example, hospital staff could engage SNF staff in a discussion about what risk factors lead to readmissions after total knee and hip replacement. They could, for instance, share an article that describes how infection control, falls, and pressure ulcers affect readmission rates for patients after knee and hip replacement so that the SNF can guide its prevention strategies toward such areas as turn schedules and fall prevention.

Providing updates on recent changes in legislation or other regulations is another common agenda item at network business meetings. For example, SNFs are typically updated when the annual financial penalties for hospital readmissions are released or when reimbursement changes are announced for post-acute care providers and continuing care. Hospitals also likely discussed the approval in both houses of Congress of the Improving Medicare Post-Acute Care Transformation (IMPACT) Act of 2014 with SNFs to ensure they understood that major changes in documentation requirements were looming in 2015.

Implement POLST, INTERACT, and Advancing Excellence Tools

SNFs that have not implemented a few basic prevention tactics should not be considered for a post-acute care network or transitional care program. Specifically, all SNFs in the post-acute care network should commit to implementing the following tools for all patients.

Physician Orders for Life-Sustaining Treatment (POLST)
A POLST form or a similar form should be completed by an SNF nurse for all patients in an SNF. Three copies should be placed in the patient's chart, and a copy should be sent each time the patient is admitted to the hospital. Rarely does the POLST form make it back to the SNF with the patient, however, so having the additional copies is critical. A POLST form typically includes information about advance directives, power of attorney, and important medications. End-of-life care goals should also be clearly stated. Most SNFs claim that they complete a POLST form for all patients, but because of the migrant nature of sick and aging patients, it is difficult to have complete compliance on POLST forms.

SNFs need to understand the importance of completing a POLST form and ensure that the form makes it to the ED with the patient 100 percent of the time. Hospital staff and case managers could focus on this tactic as a way to coordinate more effectively with SNFs. As it pertains to palliative care, the form is typically used when decisions must be made about life-sustaining treatment in the emergency room and patients equipped with a POLST form have clearly defined their desire for or against end-of-life care. Without the legal document in hand, ED doctors are often not willing to discharge the patient home.

INTERACT Tools
INTERACT (Interventions to Reduce Acute Care Transfers) tools have been widely accepted and are available online at no cost. INTERACT provides a number of effective tools:

- *Stop and Watch program:* This program empowers clinical staff to slow down and observe the patient to ensure that warning signs are not missed and patients are complying with orders and care plans.
- *SBAR:* This tool teaches caretakers to consider four steps—situation, background, assessment, and recommendation.
- *Return-to-acute-care log:* This form is used to log all patients who return to the hospital.
- *Return-to-acute-care root-cause analysis form:* This tool is used to conduct a detailed analysis of each patient who returned to the hospital and what led to the readmission.
- *Care Paths:* These are step-by-step disease-specific guides—in the form of decision trees—for nurses to determine when to call a physician and how to script the conversation. Care Paths posters should be on the wall of every SNF nursing station.

Advancing Excellence

The Advancing Excellence tool is another comprehensive tool that can be used to better track and train SNFs to avoid unnecessary hospital readmissions. In September 2006, the American Health Care Association convened a group of volunteers to develop a comprehensive tool that proved effective in a skilled-nursing environment. Now, in addition to the comprehensive quality tool, the movement has grown into collaboratives in each of the 50 states that work together to improve care transitions using the Advancing Excellence tool as a guide.

Schedule Weekly Joint Operating Committee Meetings with Each SNF

Another tactic used by post-acute care networks is scheduling weekly joint operating committee (JOC) meetings at the SNF. These meetings with SNF leadership should be attended by the ACM and the home health navigator. The meetings should last less than a half hour, have a standard agenda, and be driven for the most part by the SNF. Following is a list of suggested agenda items:

◆ *Review SNF patients.* At the weekly JOC meeting, the first agenda item is for the SNF to update the ACM and home health navigator on all patients who were transferred to the SNF and are receiving therapy. A list of all patients scheduled to be discharged in the next seven days should be reviewed, and the group should discuss the patients' postdischarge care plans and conduct home health evaluations for each patient. Often, a patient will choose the hospital-based home health agency before being discharged from the hospital. When that is the case, the home health navigator stops by the patient's room at the SNF each week to remind her that there is a plan to continue therapy in the home environment after discharge. The days of SNFs dictating which home health is selected are falling by the wayside. The hospital is now driving the entire process. Thus, after the weekly meeting concludes, the home health navigator stops by for a brief touch visit or reminder that he is looking forward to providing home health services once the SNF stay is complete.

◆ *Review follow-up care.* The meeting attendees should confirm that the SNF has scheduled a follow-up physician's office visit for all patients being discharged that week. The SNF should also confirm that each patient has transportation to and from the checkup.

◆ *Review the return-to-acute-care log.* I prefer to call this the "return to ED" log because that name emphasizes that the post-acute care provider is responsible for making sure that SNF patients do not return to the hospital by increasing communication and improving care. The SNF should have a basic understanding of every patient who left the facility to go to the hospital that week and determine if any steps could have been taken to prevent the occurrence.

- *Review root-cause analyses.* The root-cause analysis findings should be reviewed for all avoidable situations in which a patient was returned to acute care. Not all root-cause analyses need to be reviewed at each meeting. In fact, when things are working smoothly and everyone is doing what is expected on the nursing floor, return-to-acute-care cases will be rare and well controlled so that typically only one or two will need to be reviewed. However, it is critical that the SNF understands that it must complete a root-cause analysis for every patient who returns to the ED and that the findings should be available at the weekly meeting.
- *Run patient DNA tests in the SNF and share results with the hospital.* DNA reports are ordered by physicians in an SNF setting under Medicare Part B because they help the SNF reduce medication costs. Hospital-based physicians, however, are not ordering genetic testing aggressively because it is not a covered inpatient benefit. The most frequent benefits are reduced medications per patient and cost savings found in eliminating psychotropic and behavioral medications that are costly, can lessen cognitive awareness, and may increase the patient's chance of developing an infection.

  SNFs see the genetic testing as a win–win because it not only reduces their medication costs but also identifies them as a preferred provider from the hospital's perspective. The hospital can then scan a patient's genetic map into the electronic health record so that all physicians will have access to the list of medications that are most effective for that patient and at which dosages. Exhibit 9.1 (in Chapter 9) shows a typical DNA report from Vantari Genetics, a genetic testing lab in Irvine, California.
- *Review predictive software reports.* SNF facilities that want to show the hospital that they are committed to their partnership have already invested in predictive software that helps identify avoidable readmissions before they occur. Predictive software

reports also document the SNF's disease-specific readmission rate each month. These reports should be reviewed each week at the JOC meeting. (See Exhibit 3.1 in Chapter 3 for a sample report.)

♦ *Identify hospice referrals.* The SNF should be asked if any potential hospice referrals are expected in the coming days. If the hospital or accountable care organization has an affiliated hospice, it is important that post-acute care providers view the hospital-affiliated hospice as the key partner in the post-acute care network.

These are a number of tactics that can be used after discharge from the hospital. A hospital that implements them is likely to see a measurable decline in unnecessary readmissions.

REFERENCE

Tam, O. Y., S. M. Lam, H. P. Shum, C. W. Lau, K. C. Chan, and W. W. Yan. 2014. "Characteristics of Patients Readmitted to Intensive Care Unit: A Nested Case-Control Study." *Hong Kong Medical Journal* 20 (3): 194–204.

CHAPTER 5

Prevention Planning Phase Three: The Patient Returns to the Emergency Department

Although hospitals, medical groups, and health insurance companies have undertaken extensive outreach campaigns to curb high-risk patients from returning to the emergency department (ED) after discharge from the hospital, many high-risk patients continue to do so as an alternative to seeing a primary care physician or going to an urgent care clinic. Phase Three of prevention planning focuses on alternatives to the ED and tactics to follow if a patient does show up at the ED, where the goal is to avoid an unnecessary readmission to the acute care hospital.

Before reading further, it is important to understand that all of the tactics listed in Phase Three are considered to be aggressive and likely ahead of the curve. Phase Three tactics are for hospitals that are adopting a philosophy that promotes levels of care alternative to the hospital. This philosophy requires a major cultural shift on the part of organizational leadership because it is contrary to how hospitals are reimbursed. Hospitals still get paid when patients are admitted, and despite the Affordable Care Act (ACA) incentives to reduce unnecessary hospitalizations, hospital leadership remains entrenched in marketing tactics and models designed over the past 30 years to promote hospital admission. Thus, this chapter provides a look into how health systems can adapt to the new guidelines by implementing ED protocols to ensure that hospitalization is necessary.

An imperative is that the hospital and health system review how patients are currently assessed in the ED, especially because the Recovery Audit Contractor (RAC) program will require hospitals to return reimbursement dollars for patients classified as not needing acute care. Whether a patient is a readmission candidate or not, ED physicians need to ask one basic question about all patients presenting in the ED: Can this patient be cared for at a lower level of care? If the answer is yes, then the physician should stabilize the patient and begin the transfer process.

The question regarding level of patient care required is in stark contrast to the days when ED criteria for admission were more likely to focus on a different question: Can we get this patient qualified for reimbursement? What followed was lab work and orders for imaging for all patients, regardless of their reason for coming to the hospital. To use Lean or Six Sigma terminology, if your "current state" is focused on qualifying for reimbursement rather than asking if a patient could be cared for at a lower level of care, then a cultural change is needed.

Today, the "future state" is a process that assesses a patient to determine the lowest level of care necessary. Theoretically, this future state approach should already be in place because the ACA was passed in 2010 and there has been plenty of time to plan and implement.

The other critical step that needs to take place is an increased focus on studying the patient's reason for coming to the ED, especially as hospitals continue to be subject to the Emergency Medical Treatment and Active Labor Act. If the patient did not arrive via ambulance, there is a strong possibility that his reason for returning to the hospital is social and not medical. (When a patient visits the ED unnecessarily—that is, as an alternative to a physician's office visit, for a nonemergent reason, or because of patient anxiety—the ED staff call it a "social" visit.) In such cases, liability is typically the first reason an ED physician gives when defending why she erred on the side of caution and admitted a patient to the hospital who may have been in the gray area of needing readmission. Yet, if the hospital shifts its focus to determining and documenting why a patient came to the ED, there may be fewer gray areas.

For example, say a patient tells the nurse and physician, "I came to the hospital because I ran out of medication, could not afford a refill, and did not know what else to do." The medications are then refilled, and the patient is sent home. Later that evening, however, he has chest pain and returns to the ED, where it is determined that he has had a minor stroke. The family sues the hospital for discharging him home after the first visit. If the medical professionals did not ask and document the patient's reason for visiting the ED earlier in the day, the hospital is at greater risk of losing the case. However, the hospital would be in a much stronger position to defend itself if it had documented at the first ED visit that the patient only came to the ED because he ran out of medications and couldn't afford more.

I recall one ED nurse telling me that an elderly patient had come to the ED because her "tongue was dry." We have all heard similar reasons for ED visits. However, under the prior state model of simply looking to qualify the patient for reimbursement, many of these patients were admitted. Under the current state methodology of understanding the social reason for the return to the ED and admitting the patient only as a last resort (if the patient cannot be cared for at a lower level of care), patients presenting to the ED for social reasons are unlikely to be admitted.

Once a complete reprogramming of the process and a cultural shift have taken place in the ED, specifically pertaining to how patients are evaluated by physicians and case managers when determining discharge disposition, hospitals are ready to consider implementing some of the Phase Three tactics described in this chapter when a readmission candidate returns to the ED.

TRAIN MEDICARE REIMBURSEMENT EXPERTS

Many hospitals have created physician adviser positions within the ED and hospital structure and have trained them to become subject-matter experts on the criteria for patients to qualify for inpatient Medicare reimbursement. Physician advisers are often experienced hospitalists who research RAC audits and better understand what needs to be included in the documentation to demonstrate the patient's need for acute care and that his needs could not have been cared for at a lower level of care.

ESTABLISH A CALL CENTER OR HOTLINE

In the 1990s, many hospitals and health plans established nurse hotlines to counsel patients who thought they needed to return to the ED. By the early 2000s, however, most had been discontinued because there was no immediate revenue line to justify or offset the expense. Today, call centers are returning with an expanded set of services. Many organizations realize that if they can get the patient or caretaker to contact the call center rather than driving to the ED, a clinical operator with a basic set of clinical skills and knowledge will be able to direct the patient to the appropriate service and level of care for her specific situation.

These new call centers are not simply nurse hotlines. The operator may be a nurse but is just as likely to be a pharmacist, pharmacist technician, or certified nurse assistant. Most call centers today use a type of decision-tree model. Thus, when a caller contacts the center, the goal is to rule out all interventions that are billable and can drive revenue before offering any options that are expenses to the organization. As health plans offer a more comprehensive scope of post-acute care services to keep patients from unnecessary hospitalizations, the call center and decision tree become an even greater opportunity, particularly because the patient has successfully demonstrated the desired behavior of calling as opposed to going to the ED.

For example, suppose a patient calls and says, "I'm not feeling well today. I think I need to go to the ED." The operator would have a decision-tree script that allows him to drill down and identify the more specific reason for the patient's discomfort. The operator would also have a prioritized list of services that the health plan offers to its patients and would start ruling out each option until the patient and operator agree on an appropriate next step.

If the patient happens to call during business hours, the first alternative would be to refer her to her primary care physician. Thus, the call center must have a comprehensive list of physician's offices, phone numbers, and hours as well as a means to quickly contact the office to schedule an appointment. If the primary care physician is not available, the second option might be an affiliated urgent care or medical group that can serve as an alternative to the patient's primary care physician. A third option might be a visit to the post-acute care clinic (if the health system operates one). A fourth option might be to send out a home health nurse from an embedded home health partner. A fifth option might be to send a private-duty nurse, nurse practitioner, or physician assistant who is affiliated with the health plan. Each of these five options, in most cases, is a billable episode through the Medicare benefit. Thus, each option can be a revenue generator when coordinated properly. Another advantage of the decision tree is that each organization has the opportunity to prioritize the order in which it offers, and rules out, services over the telephone to each patient who calls. Top health systems also use the system to prioritize tactics that drive revenue to the organization.

Several models of call centers are available and in use, but a health system can also contract with established call centers, such as VitaPhone Health Solutions, which operates a call center in Las Vegas, Nevada, and services the entire United States. The call center provides support for remote monitoring devices from cardiology to pulmonology, in addition to the other basic services often provided by a nurse hotline. When a remote monitoring device communicates an adverse result to the command center, each specific health system has developed a model unique to its system that dictates the next steps. For example, the call may be directed to the skilled-nursing facility (SNF) or to the caretaker who is overseeing the patient. The decision tree will usually prioritize appropriate interventions that are potential revenue generators or an alternative to the ED.

The important thing to remember about the reemergence of the call center and decision tree is that the decision tree can be tailored specifically to a health plan to best meet its needs, maximize revenue opportunities, control expenses, and triage the patient in the most efficient manner. Although each health system is unique, the call center's main goal is to identify all of the different levels of care provided in that system. The next goal is to prioritize levels of care by patient need and acuity as well as by which options may be a revenue opportunity as opposed to an expense. When an organization creates an efficient model of this nature, call centers can be a solution for preventing unnecessary rehospitalization.

As noted, many health plans discontinued their call centers over the years because they were viewed as non–revenue generating and expensive. As the call center reemerges in the era of population management, however, health systems are learning that many of the options call centers can provide for patients are revenue generating or cost neutral as opposed to straight expenses.

IMPLEMENT A PARAMEDICINE APPROACH

Paramedicine is another emerging option to avoid unnecessary hospitalization. Traditionally, the role of the paramedic was to stabilize and transfer the patient to the hospital, and paramedics had a limited ability to provide care and treatment to patients. They were not authorized to provide care in the field or make care decisions for the patients. The emerging focus on paramedicine, however, turns that tradition on its head. In this new model, the term "paramedicine" describes medics who are deployed to a home setting with the intent of evaluating the patient to determine the most appropriate level of care to which to transfer her.

Before paramedicine becomes a viable option in most communities, however, a number of concerns need to be addressed because providers, specifically hospitals, are threatened by the thought of paramedicine. Hospitals fear losing revenue to this emerging service because the patients on whom hospitals relied to maintain profitability are not likely to go to the hospital in many instances. This is even more true if the paramedicine provider is not embedded in the healthcare organization or is not a preferred provider. Furthermore, reimbursement models for paramedicine are still fairly new, so beyond a few grant programs, only a few viable options are available for financing paramedicine programs.

CREATE AN ED ALERT/AWARENESS SYSTEM

The number one responsibility of hospital administration in the readmission process is alerting ED physicians, nurses, and case managers that a newly arrived patient is a potential readmission candidate. Once the administration has made the clinical team and ED physician aware, the decision to admit lies with the physician and clinical team. Although each organization takes a different approach, the following are some commonly used alert measures:

- When a patient's Social Security number is entered into the ED computer system, a text message or e-mail alert is sent if the patient has been an inpatient at that hospital in the previous 30 days.
- An electronic red flag is placed on the ED home screen alerting the nurses, physician, and ED case manager that a patient is a potential readmission candidate.

- A television monitor in the ED displays a symbol that signifies a patient is a readmission.
- The electronic or hard-copy chart is flagged with a symbol that the patient is a readmission candidate.

After serving as an acute care hospital CEO for seven years, I spent a year working as the CEO of an acute rehabilitation hospital. It was difficult switching perspectives, but from my new vantage point I set a goal of helping the local acute care hospitals prevent unnecessary readmissions. To that end, I met with the CEO of each hospital to discuss the services provided by the acute rehab hospital. I emphasized that the most important thing hospital CEOs could do was to educate staff about what to do when a readmission candidate arrives at the ED. I pointed out that the only way to hold staff accountable for the process is to make them aware that a patient is a readmission candidate, joking that "If I were still in your shoes as a hospital CEO, I would install a flashing red emergency siren inside my ED to make sure my staff are aware each time a readmission candidate returns to the hospital!" Although I may have exaggerated my potential solution, the point was made.

USE CLOUD-BASED SOFTWARE TO COMPLEMENT THE MEDICAL RECORD

As mentioned earlier, social reasons often cause high-risk Medicare fee-for-service patients to return to the ED unnecessarily. However, case-related information that would explain a patient's thought process and decision to return to the ED may not be appropriate to include in the medical record. Thus, hospitals and health systems are investing in cloud-based software packages to allow the care team to enter social commentary about a patient's care separately from the medical record.

Cloud-based data are accessible online via e-mail or the hospital website and are often accessible via the patient portal, so the patient and family members have the ability to comment on the patient's care plan any time. In the war on readmissions, the commentary and social issues described in the record may provide answers that traditional lab work and radiology procedures cannot. Health systems that have begun to use this information have found that it can play a significant role in answering questions about the patient's needs that cannot be obtained by traditional medical procedures.

PROVIDE PATIENT EDUCATION IN THE ED

Once, when I met with a group of ED physicians and staff for the first time to discuss how to handle ED patients who were readmission candidates, I was greeted with chuckles, smirks, and·whispered comments. Finally, someone asked, "Is alerting us to readmission patients and diverting them to alternative placement in the true spirit of why we are working to prevent unnecessary readmissions?"

I was glad the question had been asked and responded, "I think this is the one moment when your patient is a captive audience, so it might be the best opportunity to educate the patient on self-management techniques." Although the hospital's intent when deploying an ED case manager or nurse to the patient's bedside is to prevent unnecessary readmission, such visits provide many other benefits, so in a post-ACA model ED staff should be handling all patients in this manner.

Hospitals that have been significantly affected by Centers for Medicare & Medicaid Services RAC audits are familiar with this concept of patient education. Thus, the ED case manager should have three primary goals when meeting with a readmission candidate in the ED: identify the cause of the ED trip, educate the patient on ED alternatives, and prevent an unnecessary readmission.

Identify the Cause of the ED Trip

If the patient was not brought to the ED as the result of a 911 call, train your staff to first ask what drove the decision to come to the ED. Until the patient provides proof of a medically justified need, staff should assume that the patient's decision was not medically related and could have been made for inappropriate social reasons. This is the same type of training being done to prevent lost revenue on RAC audits. As noted, research has shown that social issues drive most readmissions to the ED with Medicare fee-for-service patients. To reiterate, the goal is to not admit any patient to the hospital who could be cared for at a lower level of care—whether or not the patient is a readmission candidate. Determining the patient's reason for coming to the ED will show what type of patient education is needed.

Educate the Patient on ED Alternatives

The time a patient spends waiting in an ED bed is a great opportunity for the case manager to pull the electronic health record, look at the patient's history, and suggest alternatives to the ED that would provide a better way to care for his healthcare needs in the future. Case managers should have a brochure or some other material describing these options. The following examples illustrate how a hospital might approach educating a patient who returns to the ED.

For example, many health systems have a post-acute care clinic designed for patients during the first three days after discharge from the hospital, SNF, or ED. A suggested talking point might be, "The medical record does not indicate that you visited our post-acute care clinic after you were discharged a few weeks ago, so I would be happy to schedule an appointment with the clinic or with your primary care physician now so you can follow up with them in the next few days." Or if the health system works closely with a home health agency, the talking point might be, "It appears that you declined a home health evaluation upon discharge a few weeks ago. May I suggest that you reconsider that decision, because an evaluation likely would have prevented your return to the ED? We strongly suggest that you allow our home health staff to visit your home and, at a minimum, go through an evaluation so you can be aware of the services they provide."

Prevent an Unnecessary Readmission

As discussed earlier, ED physicians must take a new approach when assessing patients for admission to the hospital. Although this approach is a major shift from the manner in which ED physicians have operated for the past 20 years, physicians must move forward—and not just because of readmissions. The behavior is also being driven by the RAC audits that result in Medicare's withholding payment for care that has already been provided when the patient record lacks documentation showing that the patient needed to be in the hospital.

Other steps that may be taken when the patient returns to the ED include reviewing and updating the risk assessment, reconciling medications, and inquiring about the patient's social well-being and living environment. Once again, the goal is to gather as much information as possible while the patient is in the hospital. All of that captured data should be added to the electronic health record so that a more complete snapshot of the patient and her needs is available for all caretakers now and in the future.

IDENTIFY TEACH-BACK AND MESSAGE DELIVERY OPPORTUNITIES

Patient self-management is a critical component of readmission prevention, and patient education, in turn, is a critical component of improving patient self-management. The ED provides opportunities to educate readmission candidates, and patients waiting in an ED bed are more likely to retain information than they were during their prior stay. This is particularly true if the patient has already been advised that he does not need acute inpatient hospitalization.

Thus, as discussed earlier, when an ED patient is a potential readmit, it is critical that hospitals and health systems have a defined process for educating the patient on alternatives to the ED and implement teach-back methodology. Keep in mind that the patient may be embarrassed when the education process begins and it becomes obvious that an ED visit was likely not justified. Delivering the message appropriately, with compassion and empathy, is as important as ever.

A "we are on the same team" delivery approach can be successful in sharing options to avoid the hospital. For example, the case manager might say, "In the future, we can avoid an ED visit if you call a call center, contact your primary care physician, or visit your physician or urgent care." It is also helpful to provide collateral materials the patient can take home that provide details on proper medication adherence, nutrition, hydration, exercise, and potential risk factors. Demonstrating the patient portal on a tablet can also be beneficial.

When this educational process has taken place at the bedside and medication orders have been updated and refilled if necessary, it is important to implement teach-back methodologies and have the patient repeat the instructions back. Hearing the instructions interpreted in the patient's own words and seeing it through their own actions is a proven methodology for confirming patient comprehension and preventing unnecessary readmissions.

TRANSFER THE PATIENT TO OBSERVATION STATUS

Another alternative to readmitting a patient is transferring her to observation status from the ED. Some hospitals have observation units; others commingle observation patients on the inpatient medical-surgical unit.

Hospitals often use the term *23/59*, which evolved from the original concept of observation for less than 24 hours. The term is a reminder that observation status is intended to be used for patients who need to be observed for less than 24 hours, so that a determination of admission or discharge can be made. Over the past 20 years, however, hospitals started to see an emerging trend of observation patients staying well beyond 24 hours, and observation status evolved into a holding ground or staging area for patients with no discharge disposition.

This trend created an easy opportunity for hospitals and case managers to defer efforts on patients who were difficult placements. In the past, if a case manager was handed the chart of a homeless patient, a behavioral health patient, or an elderly person with no insurance, he might just throw his hands in the air and say, "Put them on observation because no one will take them." The ACA, RAC audits, and declining hospital revenues are causing hospitals to reverse this trend and develop strict criteria for patients on observation status. All hospitals should now have specific criteria for patients being transferred to observation—readmission candidate or not—because it is a financial burden on the hospital.

Thus, although observation units and beds should be considered an alternative to inpatient admission, transferring all readmission candidates to observation status to avoid a readmission penalty for a patient is by no means a viable solution. However, if a patient's status is in question after she is assessed in the ED, observation status can be a viable last resort before admitting the patient as an inpatient.

A number of factors should be considered before transferring a patient to observation status. Cost is always a factor when transferring a patient to observation. The hospital loses money while a patient is on observation status. Although the hospital may receive significant reimbursement for an observation patient who is ultimately admitted to the hospital, updated regulations have changed how hospitals approach the observation process.

Observation patients are reimbursed at outpatient rates, which are 80 to 90 percent less than inpatient reimbursement. However, the care provided in observation is essentially the same level and expense to hospitals as inpatient care. Thus, observation should not be used as a staging ground for potentially admitting patients who do not need acute care. Traditionally, hospitals were willing to take the risk of transferring patients to observation status in hopes that they would eventually transfer to inpatient by default, but as mentioned, the financial implications of using observation as an alternative to readmission is likely more costly in the long run than if the patient were readmitted as an inpatient. Remember, hospitals are reimbursed for patients who qualify as readmissions, but they are penalized at the end of the year on the basis of their comparative readmission rate of Medicare fee-for-service patients.

TRANSFER THE PATIENT DIRECTLY FROM THE ED TO A LONG-TERM ACUTE CARE HOSPITAL OR ACUTE REHABILITATION FACILITY

One of the best-kept secrets in readmission prevention is that patients who need acute care but would qualify as readmission candidates can be transferred directly from the ED to a long-term acute care (LTAC) hospital or an inpatient rehabilitation facility (IRF). Both LTAC hospitals and IRFs (better known as acute rehab facilities) are licensed by the state as acute hospitals so they can care for very sick patients. This would also be true for LTAC unit (or licensed "hospital in hospital") arrangements or inpatient rehab units within the hospital, assuming that each unit has a Medicare provider number separate from the acute hospital's.

Why is this a secret? Did you know LTAC hospitals have an intensive care unit? Did you know LTAC hospitals have full-service operating rooms? In essence, if a patient who returns to your ED is identified as a readmission candidate and it is determined that he needs acute care or surgery, the hospital could stabilize and transfer him from the ED directly to an LTAC hospital to avoid the patient's counting toward the readmission penalty. This may be the largest loophole available to acute providers in the readmission penalty process.

Another well-kept secret about IRFs is that patients can be admitted directly from home. A three-day inpatient hospital stay is not required, nor is the patient required to have been in the hospital in the prior 30 days. The only real requirement for a Medicare patient to be admitted to an IRF is a physician order. For this reason, patients are commonly admitted to an IRF directly from a physician's office, urgent care clinic, assisted-living facility, or home. For the most part, getting a physician's order from an IRF facility medical director can be as easy as having the facility liaison or nurse call the physician and say, "We just received a call from the ED, and they have a patient who needs acute rehab. Could you please write an order?"

Although direct-from-ED transfer to LTAC hospitals and IRFs remains a rarely used tactic, progressive health systems are using these levels of post-acute care as a key strategy in their population management plan. For example, in 2013, UCLA Health System and Cedars-Sinai Medical Center announced a joint venture to purchase a recently shuttered hospital in Los Angeles and converted it to an acute rehabilitation hospital.

TRANSFER THE PATIENT DIRECTLY FROM THE ED TO AN SNF

Transfers from the ED directly to an SNF have been gaining momentum in recent years and are a good choice when the patient does not need acute care but cannot safely return home. To qualify for the Medicare benefit in the SNF, however, the patient must have spent three consecutive midnights as an inpatient in an acute care setting in the past 30 days.

This requirement has been the subject of much recent debate. Many argue that the three-midnight requirement is no longer appropriate because it is a barrier in a population management delivery model. With the significant increase in hospital observation days and updated requirements that observation days cannot be converted to inpatient days, the three-midnight requirement remains controversial as we migrate toward a true population management delivery system.

The debate about SNFs has a positive component, however. Let's compare the definition of a readmission candidate to the Medicare three-midnight requirement for SNFs:

◆ Readmission candidate
  – A Medicare fee-for-service patient
  – Discharged from an acute care hospital in the prior 30 days
  – If readmitted to any acute care hospital within 30 days of discharge from the index stay, the hospital that cared for the patient during her index stay is penalized
◆ Qualifying hospital stay for Medicare SNF benefit
  – A Medicare fee-for-service patient
  – Discharged from an acute care hospital in the prior 30 days
  – Had a minimum stay of three midnights as an inpatient in an acute care setting

With most hospital length-of-stay averages exceeding three days, any patient who returns to the ED within 30 days of discharge (and is a readmission candidate) will likely qualify for the SNF Medicare benefit if transferred directly to an SNF. This is a tremendous opportunity for SNFs.

Hospitals have seen an increase in direct-from-ED transfers in recent years, and this trend will continue as hospitals continue to incur reduced reimbursement as a result of RAC audits recovering funds for patients who did not meet acute care requirements. The biggest obstacle is educating ED physicians on the opportunity and the scope of services that SNFs provide.

As mentioned before, to best train ED physicians to stabilize and transfer patients to lower levels of care, a cultural shift is likely necessary. Thus, the hospital and health system must first alert the ED physicians and staff in real time when the patient is a 30-day readmission candidate. This can be done with text or e-mail alerts. Once the administration has fulfilled its responsibility of creating a process to alert the ED staff, the burden of responsibility to avoid the readmission passes to the ED physicians and case managers who ultimately determine the patient's discharge disposition.

This cultural shift requires a major retraining of ED case managers who by practice have primarily prioritized transferring or discharging patients out of the ED as quickly as possible in the past. Regardless of the direction given by administration, as a result of industry pressures and standards pertaining to ED wait times and the additional paperwork involved in patient transfers, it has become second nature for case managers and ED physicians to choose the quickest option to empty the bed, or the path of least resistance in determining the patient's discharge disposition. This type of behavior became embedded in hospital culture in recent years and contributed to the creation of RAC audits and penalties for admitting patients who did not need acute care.

Another issue is that ED physicians are not always aware of the capabilities of SNFs. The ED physicians at one client hospital of mine did not know the scope of services provided by each SNF in the community, and this lack of knowledge was a significant impediment to their ability to write a direct-to-SNF transfer and have the confidence that it would be seamless. Within 24 hours I asked each of the SNFs in the network to complete the INTERACT SNF capabilities form. We then consolidated each of the seven SNFs' capabilities onto a single form, laminated it, and posted it in the ED. We included the 24-hour contact line for each SNF to facilitate transfers around the clock.

Once the capabilities spreadsheet was posted, we educated the SNFs that they needed to be prepared to accept patients for immediate transfer at all hours and on weekends. When considering a patient for admission, the SNF admission process (much like those for LTAC hospitals and IRFs) is based on three primary criteria:

1. Do the patient's clinical needs fall within the facility's scope of services?
2. Does the patient have insurance so the facility can be reimbursed for the care provided?
3. Does the patient have a predetermined discharge destination, or could this patient become a difficult discharge that would get stuck in the facility beyond the days needed to recover (while the facility no longer gets reimbursed for those days)?

Thus, the directive to the SNFs for accepting readmission candidates who would be direct-from-ED transfers is simple: The on-site nurse at the SNF needs to be empowered to accept patients 24/7 on the basis of their clinical needs. Once that authorization is received, the patient transfer should be scheduled because the SNF often is not able to confirm during nonbusiness hours that the patient has available Medicare SNF days. The message from the hospital to SNFs in a post-ACA model should be simple: Approve the patient transfer immediately so that we can clear the bed in our ED, or else we will call another SNF that will gladly accept Medicare patients and take the chance that they have available days to cover their SNF stay.

Without a quick, simple process to facilitate direct transfers from the ED to an SNF, LTAC hospital, or IRF, it is unlikely that ED physicians, nurses, and case managers will change their existing tactics of clearing the ED bed as quickly as possible. The administration is responsible for ensuring that these steps and cultural changes take place so that the hospital does not suffer financially as a result of the bad habits developed in the ED during the fee-for-service era. If the C-suite does not take a stand and develop a firm plan that involves the ED's migration toward a population management model, these bad, financially burdensome, path-of-least-resistance patient flow habits developed in the ED will continue.

Part III

TRANSITIONAL CARE PROGRAMS AND MODELS

CHAPTER 6

Transitional Care Programs and Models

Many hospitals address the readmissions problem by implementing a process often referred to as a "transitional care program." However, that term is somewhat of a misnomer; although transitional care programs are a key component of reducing readmissions, they are designed more to support the population management models that were envisioned with the creation of the Affordable Care Act. Still, transitional care programs also employ many of the tactics used in the readmission prevention planning phases discussed in Part II.

A detailed description of available transitional care programs would fill an entire book and is outside the scope of this book's focus on readmission issues. Still, readers should become familiar with the most common transitional care programs, so brief descriptions of the programs that affect readmission prevention are presented here.

According to the National Transitions of Care Coalition (NTOCC 2011), there are seven essential intervention categories, which are found in different combinations in transitional care programs:

1. Medications management
2. Transition planning

3. Patient and family engagement and education
4. Information transfer
5. Follow-up care
6. Healthcare provider engagement
7. Shared accountability across providers and organizations

Transitional care models are templates, and hospitals and health systems tweak them to best suit local needs. When developing your hospital's readmission prevention strategy, keep in mind that no two hospitals or communities are identical. Thus, your program should not be identical to the program at another facility, no matter how successful that program proved to be.

CARE TRANSITIONS INTERVENTIONS

The evidence-based Care Transitions Interventions (CTI) model, often called the *Coleman Model* because it is based on research by Dr. Eric Coleman, focuses on four pillars:

1. Medication self-management
2. Dynamic patient-centered record
3. Follow-up
4. Red flags

CTI calls its ambulatory case managers "transition coaches." The transition coaches use many of the tactics described in the three prevention planning phases and has the goal of getting the patient to take responsibility for his own care during the transition from acute care to home (Coleman, Rosenbek, and Roman 2013).

Each of the four pillars emphasizes patient education, accountability, and self-management. The patient education process begins with making sure the patient understands her medication regimen and how each medication affects the body. Patient education and engagement remain the focus with a dynamic, comprehensive, patient-centered record because it is critical that the patient takes responsibility for sharing it with her physician. The patient is also educated on the importance of the follow-up visit, what health-related warning signs or red flags are important, and how to respond to a red flag. More information about CTI is available at www.caretrasnsitions.org.

PROJECT BOOST

Project BOOST (Better Outcomes for Older Adults through Safe Transitions), developed by the Society of Hospital Medicine (SHM), provides mentoring by subject-matter experts and a tool kit for improving discharge. The tools and instructions include screening and assessment tools, discharge checklists, teach-back protocols, written discharge instructions, and transition records.

BOOST's comprehensive risk assessment is formed around the "8Ps" (SHM 2014c):

1. Problems with medications
2. Psychological
3. Principal diagnosis
4. Physical limitations
5. Poor health literacy
6. Poor social support
7. Prior hospitalization
8. Palliative care

BOOST also includes a 72-hour follow-up call for high-risk patients.

CTI and BOOST have several similarities. In fact, Dr. Eric Coleman was the advisory board chair for the Project BOOST team. Like CTI, BOOST focuses heavily on patient engagement—using teach-back methods and sending a medication list home with the patient. Also, BOOST mentors play a role similar to that of coaches in the CTI model.

The two programs outline distinctly different responsibilities, however. BOOST is a formal program structured to provide nine months of training and preparation for mentors before launch of a site and continued individualized mentoring after the launch. BOOST also relies on a community collaborative and a team to support the process. In 2013, more than 25 Project BOOST sites and programs were in use nationwide, and the BOOST California Collaborative was working to launch 20 sites by the end of 2014.

For sites implementing BOOST, the average readmission rate decreased from 14.2 percent to 11.2 percent (Nagamine 2011). Although a 3 percent decrease may seem trivial, several sites had significant improvements. St. Mary's Hospital in St. Louis, Missouri, had a 42 percent decrease in 30-day readmissions (SHM 2014b), and at Piedmont Hospital in Atlanta, Georgia, the readmission rate dropped 17 percent for those under age 70 after implementing BOOST (SHM 2014a). More information about Project BOOST and how to apply to become a mentored site is available at www .hospitalmedicine.org/BOOST/.

PROJECT RED

Project RED (Re-Engineered Discharge), developed at Boston University Medical Center under the leadership of Brian Jack, MD, is a standardized discharge intervention that includes patient education, expanded discharge planning, and postdischarge telephone follow-up reinforcement. The model focuses on reengineering patient discharge by standardizing the process to make sure patients are prepared to go home.

Project RED focuses more on postdischarge follow-up than do some of the other models. Boston University Medical Center studied the discharge process in detail and created an evidenced-based program. Although Project RED still emphasizes patient education and preparation for discharge, postdischarge follow-up for high-risk patients is also a great concern, so the program includes a follow-up call at 24 to 48 hours, confirmation that a follow-up physician appointment was scheduled, and confirmation that the patient kept the postdischarge physician appointment. According to Shagofa Zamon, Project RED coordinator at St. Rose Hospital in San Ramon, California, the three keys to a successful Project RED program are building a good rapport with patients, making effective follow-up phone calls, and keeping enrollment numbers high. He said that St. Rose's 30-day readmission rate dropped from 11.9 percent to 8 percent, and its 90-day readmission rate dropped from 21 percent to 14 percent within the initial 12 months of launching Project RED. St. Rose also conducted extensive education programs with its local skilled-nursing facilities.

BRIDGE MODEL

The Bridge Model, also known as the *Enhanced Discharge Planning Program*, is telephone based and focuses on three phases: predischarge, postdischarge, and 30-day follow-up (www.transitionalcare .org). Bridge care coordinators (BCCs) serve as ambulatory case managers for seniors as they transition home from the hospital. In the Bridge Model, a biophysical evaluation is conducted before and after the patient is discharged to identify barriers to a safe transition home and develop a plan to address specific obstacles to the patient's safety in his home environment.

Before discharge, the BCC reviews the patient's electronic health record, attends interdisciplinary rounds at the hospital, and meets with the patient and family. One of the more unique attributes of the Bridge Model is that the BCCs conduct an in-person postdischarge assessment to identify any new challenges or needs that have arisen since the patient returned to her usual living environment.

The BCCs are a support system connecting the patient with the necessary providers and resources throughout the first 30 days after the hospital episode. They also serve as patient advocates and provide positive reinforcement. At 30 days postdischarge, the BCC telephones the patient to make sure he remains stable and that there are no new challenges or threats to the patient's continued rehabilitation and well-being.

Much like several of the other transitional care programs, the Bridge Model emphasizes data collection and quality improvement to ensure quality outcomes. One study suggests that Bridge participants had a readmission rate of 19.5 percent, compared with a rate of 26.0 percent for the control group of nonparticipants (Rosenberg 2013). By 2013, the Bridge Model had been implemented in six sites in the Community-Based Care Transition Program (a federally funded grant program that provides financial support for care transitions) and at least 20 other communities nationwide (Golden 2013).

MEDICATION REACH

The Medication REACH (Reconciliation, Education, Access, Counseling, Healthy Patient at Home) program, pioneered by Einstein Healthcare Network, focuses on medication adherence (for a full summary, see the case example in Appendix B). Case managers and social workers identify patients they believe to be at high risk for readmission and recommend them for the program. Some of the tools used to ensure adherence include a personalized pictorial chart, a weekly medicine box, and personal patient coaching and counseling before and after discharge. Following are the program's tenets:

◆ *Reconciliation:* A pharmacist or pharmaceutical technician confirms the accuracy of the patient's medications before discharge.
◆ *Education:* A pharmacist or pharmaceutical technician meets with the patient to ensure that she understands the medication regimen.

- *Access:* The hospital ensures that the patient has a 30-day supply of medication after discharge, regardless of her ability to pay.
- *Counseling:* The pharmacist meets with the patient on the day of discharge and telephones her several days before the end of the 30-day postdischarge period to ensure compliance.
- *Healthy patient at home:* The ultimate goal of the program is to ensure the patient's health and well-being at home.

Einstein estimates that each patient readmission costs approximately $7,200 (LaPiene 2014). Einstein also notes that up to 50 percent of patients do not take medications as prescribed and that many patients are readmitted as a result of improper medication adherence.

In 2013, REACH received a hospital best-practice award from the American Society of Health-System Pharmacists and the American Pharmacists Association for reducing its hospital readmission and medication usage rates (Remstein and Perry 2013).

POST-ACUTE CARE TRANSITIONS (PACT)

Post-Acute Care Transitions (PACT) is a home-visit program developed for Kaiser Permanente Colorado by Jodi Smith, MSN, who previously served as the lead interventionist on Dr. Eric Coleman's CTI research team. PACT features a one-time home visit by an advanced practice nurse within 72 hours of discharge from the acute care hospital.

High-risk patients are identified in the hospital and recommended for PACT. These patients are provided with evidence-based, post-acute care transitional clinical and educational support. The two primary goals are readmission prevention and identification of postdischarge medication discrepancies. The postdischarge visit includes the following:

- Physical assessment
- Comprehensive medication reconciliation
- Education on the medication regimen
- Care plan modifications as needed
- Identification of needed resources in the home
- Customized disease management education tools

Since implementing PACT, Kaiser Permanente Colorado has seen notable improvement in fulfilling the National Committee for Quality Assurance quality measures pertaining to transitions of care. PACT has become a popular model with many other hospitals nationwide in recent years.

TRANSITIONAL CARE MODEL

Developed at the University of Pennsylvania by Mary Naylor, PhD, RN, the Transitional Care Model (TCM) uses a multidisciplinary team led by a transitional care nurse with a master's degree. The team focuses on treating chronically ill high-risk seniors. Like many of the other transitional care programs, TCM calls for interventions before, during, and after discharge from the hospital. In 2013, the Coalition for Evidence-Based Policy recognized TCM as a "top-tier" evidence-based approach for its demonstrated quality improvements and healthcare savings (*Managed Care* 2014).

The University of Pennsylvania has a long history of research on transitional care and was conducting studies on value-based care delivery and prevention of avoidable readmissions long before the Affordable Care Act and its readmission penalties. In addition to TCM, the University of Pennsylvania is home to the RightCare Solutions software developed by Dr. Kathryn Bowles, which is regarded as the leading risk-stratification software on the market. The software is known for its short, user-friendly questionnaire that can be administered by nurses or case managers in the emergency department or on admission to the hospital and that accurately predicts the patient's post-acute care risk factor. The program also links the hospital to post-acute care providers who can contribute to the ongoing risk assessment.

OTHER PROGRAMS

Several other transitional care programs have been implemented with great success:

- Geriatric Resources for Assessment and Care of Elders (GRACE), Indiana University
- The Guided Care Model, Johns Hopkins University
- Home-based Primary Care, US Department of Veterans Affairs
- State Action on Avoidable Rehospitalizations (STAAR), Institute for Healthcare Improvement

SUMMARY

Although each of the programs described in this chapter has unique attributes, the programs share a number of constants:

- Risk stratification to identify high-risk patients
- Patient engagement
- Interventions before, during, and after discharge
- Consistent communication
- Medication management and patient comprehension of medication regimen
- Patient education
- Ambulatory case management (via a navigator, coach, or similar position)
- Post-acute care follow-up
- 30-day follow-up (often by telephone)

These are the factors to consider as you determine the transitional care coordination and readmission prevention strategy that best fits the unique needs of your organization. The following Perspective describes how use of placement services can reduce readmissions by helping discharge planners identify the best transitional care strategy.

PERSPECTIVE
Advantages of Using Placement Services to Help Reduce Hospital Readmissions

By Chuck Bongiovanni
CEO, CarePatrol Franchise Systems

Discharging patients to the proper care environment is critical to hospitals seeking to lower readmission rates, but because the proper care environment varies according to the patient, social workers or discharge planners may find it challenging to make the determination. One particular patient category with high readmission rates is elderly patients with multiple chronic conditions. The patient profile will dictate the most appropriate discharge environment, which may be one of three options:

1. Home
2. Nursing home
3. Assisted-living or memory care community

When a patient is discharged to home (with or without supportive services), the discharge decision must, but too often does not, consider the capabilities of the spouse or identified caregiver. For example, it may be medically appropriate to discharge an 85-year-old patient home after a heart attack, but his 82-year-old spouse may not be prepared physically or emotionally to take on such a demanding responsibility.   →

Stressed spouses and family members may not share their concerns with the hospital discharge planner because of feelings of loyalty or obligation. For this reason, patients and caregivers should be educated on the respite option assisted-living communities can offer.

Determining which specific assisted-living community or nursing home would provide the safest discharge environment for that patient is a daunting task. Knowing all the available options is key to successfully completing this task, but realistically, no social worker or discharge planner working full-time in a hospital can stay current on all the options in the area. The solution is simple: Placement agencies are excellent resources. They serve as extensions of the social worker in the community and are local experts on assisted-living community and nursing home options. Because placement agencies focus on local housing options for seniors, they possess expert knowledge regarding the quality and capability of each housing option to care for specific chronic conditions.

A note of caution: Do not confuse placement agencies with referral agencies. Referral agencies only offer families a list of options available in the community. In contrast, placement agencies meet personally with the patient and their family to

- evaluate the patient's care needs,
- review available financial resources, and
- understand the patient's personal preferences.

With this care evaluation, the agency is able to identify the most appropriate assisted-living community or nursing home.

$\rightarrow$

After the care evaluation, a good agency personally arranges for and accompanies the family on a tour of recommended facilities and helps them in the decision-making process. The service is provided at no cost to the hospital, patient, or family. Instead, the assisted-living community pays a fee to the agency after a senior moves into the facility.

In summary, hospital social workers and discharge planners do not have time to visit every assisted-living community or keep up to date on their care and violation histories. That is where the expertise and personalized services of a placement agency become priceless and help ensure that the patient is placed in a care environment that will minimize the risk of readmission.

The usual hospital practice of giving patients and their families a list of senior housing options requires the patient and family to execute a search on their own. Because they have limited time and knowledge and are under considerable stress, they tend to choose a site on the basis of appearance or convenience rather than the facility's ability to provide appropriate care for the senior. Hence, too many seniors are readmitted—and these readmissions could have been avoided.

In contrast, hospitals that are effectively responding to the readmission crisis are leveraging the services of placement agencies. The use of placement agencies to identify post-hospitalization care options

- reduces hospital readmission rates,
- enables timely discharges,
- assists in difficult discharges,
- decreases workload stress for social workers and discharge planners, and
- reduces patient and family stress.

REFERENCES

Coleman, E., S. Rosenbek, and S. Roman. 2013. "Disseminating Evidence-Based Care into Practice." *Population Health Management* 16 (4): 227–34.

Golden, R. 2013. "Bridge Model Decreases Readmissions Through Segmented Follow-ups." *National Transitions of Care Coalition Impact Newsletter*, Fall. http://cmi-ntocc .informz.net/CMI-NTOCC/data/images/documents /impactaug2013.pdf.

LaPiene, B. 2014. "Einstein's Comprehensive Unit-Based Safety Program." *Population Health News* 27 (2): 7.

Managed Care. 2014. "A Conversation with Mary D. Naylor, PhD, RN: Managing the Transition from the Hospital." Published June. http://managedcaremag.com/archives /2014/6/conversation-mary-d-naylor-phd-rn-managing -transition-hospital.

Nagamine, J. 2011. "Project BOOST." Presentation. Avoid Readmissions Through Collaboration. Accessed October 25, 2014. www.avoidreadmissions.com/wwwroot/userfiles /documents/22/arc-project-boost.pdf.

National Transitions of Care Coalition (NTOCC). 2011. "Care Transition Bundle: Seven Essential Intervention Categories." Posted February 7. www.ntocc.org/Portals/0/PDF /Compendium/SevenEssentialElements.pdf.

Remstein, R., and R. Perry. 2013. "The Trenton Health Team." *Readmission News* 2 (9): 1. www.trentonhealthteam.org/tht /readmissions0913PerryRemstein.pdf.

Rosenberg, W. 2013. "Implementing the Bridge Model to Reduce Readmissions at a Major Medical Center." Presentation at the California Readmission Summit, San Francisco, October 10.

www.avoidreadmissions.com/wwwroot/userfiles/documents
/246/walter-rosenberg-implementing-the-bridge-model.pdf.

Society of Hospital Medicine (SHM). 2014a. "BOOSTing a
Team Approach to Patient Care." Project BOOST case study,
Piedmont Hospital, Atlanta, Georgia. Accessed October 25.
https://store.hospitalmedicine.org/Web/Quality___
Innovation/Mentored_Implementation/Project_BOOST
/BOOST_Preliminary_Results_from_Pilot_Sites.aspx.

———. 2014b. "Reducing Readmissions and So Much More."
Project BOOST case study, St. Mary's Hospital, St. Louis,
Missouri. Accessed October 25. https://store.hospital
medicine.org/Web/Quality___Innovation/Mentored
_Implementation/Project_BOOST/BOOST_Preliminary
_Results_from_Pilot_Sites.aspx.

———. 2014c. "Touch Points: Admission, During Hospitalization, and Discharge." Risk Assessment–8P Project BOOST
implementation toolkit. Accessed October 25. www.hospital
medicine.org/Web/Quality_Innovation/Implementation
_Toolkits/Project_BOOST/Web/Quality___Innovation
/Implementation_Toolkit/Boost/BOOST_Intervention
/Tools/Risk_Assessment.aspx.

Part IV

READMISSION PREVENTION MODELS BY LEVEL OF CARE

Readmission Prevention Tactics for Hospitals: Developing a Hospital Readmission Plan

The goal of this chapter is to provide acute care hospital executives with a road map for strategizing and developing an effective readmission prevention plan for their hospital. First, civic goals for developing the plan will be identified—goals beyond merely avoiding readmission penalties from the Centers for Medicare & Medicaid Services (CMS). Second, specific focus areas will be identified for different types of hospitals, including rural hospitals, urban hospitals, health systems, academic and teaching hospitals, safety-net hospitals, and critical-access hospitals.

FOUR OVERALL GOALS IN DEVELOPING A READMISSION PREVENTION PLAN

Although the readmission penalties implemented by CMS in the Affordable Care Act (ACA) have prompted organizations to form work groups to address the preventable readmission problem, organizations committed to value-based care look beyond the penalties and aim for a true population health management strategy. With that in mind, you should identify your organization's objectives and priorities before starting to develop a readmission prevention plan.

All hospitals should consider the following goals when developing a readmission prevention plan:

1.   Admit only inpatients who cannot be cared for at a lower level of care.
2.   Create a health information exchange (HIE) that is accessible to all community providers and caretakers.
3.   Reduce improper admissions that lead to Recovery Audit Contractor (RAC) audit denials.
4.   Reduce preventable readmissions and resulting penalties from CMS.

Goal 1: Admit Only Inpatients Who Cannot Be Cared for at a Lower Level of Care

The ACA aims to position the hospital as the last resort in providing care to patients and keeping them well. When hospitals begin viewing themselves as the last resort in the new post-ACA delivery model, then and only then will they have clarity in designing an effective readmissions prevention program. The name of the game is not *readmission* prevention—it is *admission* prevention. That concept is a tough pill for hospitals to swallow because they are still reimbursed almost entirely for putting "heads in beds."

Thus, implementing an effective readmission prevention program will require hospitals to implement criteria for inpatient admissions that rule out all lower levels of care when evaluating a patient in the emergency department (ED). This is a different approach for ED physicians than the methodology of the past, which, in short, was to run a series of tests and look for any reason to admit a patient to justify billing for reimbursement.

The ACA incentivizes hospitals and insurers to better coordinate care and prevent unnecessary hospital admissions. Note that it is prevent *admissions*, not *readmissions*. The goal is to make sure the right patients are being admitted at all times, not just when they are 30-day readmission candidates. Thus, it is important to have strict, up-to-date inpatient admission criteria that limit a hospital's liability and exposure to RAC audits and resulting reimbursement recovery from CMS.

If hospitals strive to admit only patients who cannot be cared for at a lower level of care, they will benefit from the financial incentives created by the ACA. In turn, an effective admission program solves the problems of readmission and a hospital's exposure to lost revenue in the RAC audit process.

Goal 2: Create a Health Information Exchange That Is Accessible to All Community Providers and Caretakers

In 1996, HIPAA (the Health Insurance Portability and Accountability Act) was implemented as a means of ensuring privacy when exchanging personal health information. Just 13 years later, however, the passage of the ACA began a push for online universal information exchange—that is, online patient portals that are accessible to all caregivers and providers. Although access to personal health information will still require the patient's authorization, this authorization will likely allow more sharing with relevant parties.

The most effective way to make care decisions about a patient is by having an abundance of information about his individual history. This is particularly true in an evolving delivery model where the inpatient physicians are not the patients' primary care physicians but rather hospitalists and skilled-nursing specialists who are unfamiliar with the patients they are treating. Ultimately, a comprehensive HIE that includes electronic health record data and cloud-based (similar to text messaging) conversational data and that stores both permanently at all points of care will become a physician's best resource. Keep in mind that under the new model, the delivery system also includes providers focused on wellness and healthy lifestyles. Thus, the portal would store input and data from all caretakers, including

- the hospital,
- doctor's office,
- nursing home,
- ancillary provider,
- assisted-living staff,
- pharmacist,
- home health provider,
- private duty nurse,
- senior center wellness caregiver,
- adult day care provider,
- healthy lifestyle providers (e.g., fitness gym), and
- individual patient and family input.

By having extensive pertinent data available to caretakers at every step, particularly in the ED, physicians can make more informed care decisions based on the patient's personal history and immediate needs as opposed to a reimbursement model that no longer exists. In the old model, ED physicians relied almost entirely on the patient's input and social justification for visiting the ED. For instance, a patient could say she is having pain in her abdomen, and the physician would run tests on the basis of that information and then decide whether to admit her as an inpatient. Today, an HIE would provide the physician with additional information about the patient—and in an era where data rule, there can never be enough information when making an important decision. The importance of data is never clearer than when a patient visits the ED and a physician needs to decide whether to admit her to the hospital as an acute care inpatient.

Goal 3: Reduce Improper Admissions That Lead to RAC Audit Denials

If an organization does an effective job of implementing a system for Goals 1 and 2, then the goal of reducing improper admissions that lead to RAC audit denials will be easily accomplished. By making those two operational changes, an organization will be well positioned to minimize the risk that it will have to return reimbursement funds to the federal government.

Goal 4: Reduce Preventable Readmissions and Resulting Penalties from CMS

Much like Goal 3, if an organization does an effective job of implementing a system for Goals 1 and 2, then the goal of reducing preventable readmissions will be within reach. As discussed earlier, the true approach in the new healthcare delivery system is preventing avoidable admissions. Hospitals must implement protocols that ensure that patients who can be cared for at a lower level of care are not admitted as inpatients. Then a hospital will be well positioned to maximize financial efficiencies and reduce exposure to readmission penalties.

SAMPLE STEPS IN PLANNING AND IMPLEMENTING A READMISSION PREVENTION PLAN

Once your organization has successfully identified goals, which would likely include some or all four of those listed here, the team can begin the necessary steps to develop a hospital-specific program for your organization. In some cases, the program might have more of a community focus, if appropriate for the stakeholders involved. However, keep in mind that the hospital is the only entity subject to readmission penalties and therefore should take a leading role in the work group.

In the future, organizations will move closer to a patient-centered care model, which will widen the focus from readmission prevention to population health management. If done properly, your work group should be able to address both issues with the same solutions. Following is a list of simple steps in planning and implementing your readmission prevention plan. Although organizations may choose to implement multiple tactics listed in this chapter, the tactics were written as individual approaches, so implementing all of them is not necessary.

- *Form a team or work group.* Keep the team small but be sure to include the chief nursing officer or chief operating officer. The director of case management must also take an active role because if the case management and social services team does not support the changes, implementation is doomed to fail. A member of the information technology team should also be included in the work group.
- *Develop an effective implementation plan.* Your team's hours of work could be wasted if the organization does not develop an effective implementation plan. This process should start as soon as the work group is formed by making sure major stakeholders are involved from the get-go. If possible, the CEO should champion the effort because the entire leadership team needs to be behind it. If she is not in complete support, the entire plan is likely to fail. The team leader could be another high-ranking member of the administrative team, preferably the chief nursing officer or chief operating officer. Some organizations choose the chief strategy officer or vice president of post-acute care services to lead these efforts but run into roadblocks when changes start affecting inpatient operations, which is why involving the chief nursing officer

in the work group from the beginning is critical. Others have appointed the director of case management to lead these efforts but have learned that even when the director of case management is widely respected in the organization, someone from the administrative team needs to champion the readmission prevention effort or it will face operational roadblocks at some point.

- *Establish clear goals.* The work group's goals will often be identified by the administrative team but may be delegated to the work group. In any case, it is wise to start with the four goals identified earlier in this chapter and build from there by adding further goals if necessary.
- *Implement an HIE and/or electronic health record.* Connectivity and access to information are critical in developing an effective readmission prevention plan and population management strategy. The first goal is to collect all the data you can while the patient is in the hospital. The second goal is to connect as many community providers as possible so you have as much information as possible at your fingertips if the patient returns to the ED.
- *Alert your team when a potential readmission shows up.* When it comes to pure readmission prevention, the administration's main role is to alert ED physicians and staff (as soon as possible via text or e-mail) when a patient is a readmission candidate per CMS penalty guidelines.
- *Evaluate inpatient admission criteria for all ED patients.* Having appropriate criteria for inpatient admissions—specifically, by ruling out the possibility that the patient's needs could be met at a lower level of care—is the most effective tactic in running an efficient hospital. In addition, it will allow you to minimize unnecessary readmissions.
- *Establish, implement, and operate an ED case management system.* The hospital's ED case managers must take an active role in any readmission prevention plan and must support the process for it to succeed.

- *Prioritize patient education.* Patient self-management is the single most effective way to solve the readmission problem. Consistent patient education is the most efficient way to improve self-management. The importance of self-management will be discussed in greater detail later in the book.
- *Use internal resources.* The ultimate objective of an organization and business is to develop and maintain a profitable business structure. Regardless of an organization's mission, if it does not remain profitable, it cannot continue to operate. With that in mind, as your work group assembles the readmission prevention plan, focus on business opportunities and new revenue streams. Organizations that have a home health agency or skilled-nursing facility (SNF), including an SNF distinct part (an SNF unit or subacute care unit located within the walls of an acute hospital), are well positioned to generate additional revenue while improving their ability to manage the patient outside of the acute care setting. In fact, home health is the one entity that allows a hospital to monitor a patient in the home while still being reimbursed for delivering healthcare services.
- *Consider community resources.* All community resources should be considered when developing a readmission prevention plan. Community resources might include transportation, adult day programs, and access to grants. Some hospitals have included representatives from community resources on their work team. However, invitations to people outside the hospital should be discussed. The goal of the hospital work group is to develop a plan that meets the needs of the hospital and the patients it serves. When outside representatives are included in the work group, the clarity of objectives may be compromised and goals, even when clearly outlined, may be influenced and questioned by the outside parties.
- *Explore technology solutions.* Technology solutions for managing patients outside of the hospital are developing rapidly. Genetic testing, for instance, is an emerging way to improve patient care, reduce medication errors and costs, and give

physicians and pharmacists a specific game plan that best meets each patient's needs. Personal DNA mapping, which is covered under Medicare Part B, is becoming imperative for patient care. Remote monitoring, another technological innovation, allows hospitals to discharge patients home sooner while still being able to monitor them around the clock from a skilled-nursing, assisted-living, or home environment. Remote monitoring capabilities were previously limited to intensive care or telemetry units in acute care hospitals. Hospitals should not delay in implementing such technologies—not only do they reduce the cost of healthcare delivery and improve care, but they are also reimbursed in many cases.

◆ *Communicate options for follow-up.* One of the most critical issues in patient education is making sure patients know what their options are if they experience pain or discomfort after discharge and wonder if they should return to the hospital. Ensuring that the patient understands the proper telephone numbers to call, including the primary care physician's office, urgent care clinic, follow-up clinics, ancillary providers, senior centers, or other practitioners at different levels, is one of the most critical factors in avoiding unnecessary readmissions. The hospital needs to go to great lengths to make sure the patient knows what his options are other than returning to the ED.

◆ *Identify new revenue streams.* The ACA was a big blow to hospitals in terms of profitability. The balance of power in the delivery system shifted even further away from hospitals and physicians and gave more influence to health plans and insurers. The changing delivery model has already resulted in lower admissions nationwide and will continue to affect profitability as hospitals receive less reimbursement as a result of lower censuses. Many hospitals that have been successful are now faced with the challenge of identifying new revenue streams to survive. As your team develops your readmission prevention plan, profitability and new revenue streams should be at the forefront of every decision made.

- *Have measurable goals.* The work group should clearly identify and communicate measurable goals to the whole organization, along with the importance of the initiatives, timeline, and how the program's success is anticipated to affect the organization. This message should be repeated and updated regularly—monthly, or at a minimum quarterly—so that the entire organization can be kept up to date on the success of the implementation. As always, objectives should be measurable.

Although this list of recommended steps to develop an effective readmission prevention plan is by no means complete, it serves as a viable template or starting point for any organization, along with the specific tactics to implement for each phase described in Chapters 3–5. These four chapters should be consulted when you select the tactics to be implemented for your hospital-specific readmission prevention plan. In addition, the Perspective at the end of this chapter describes how improved communication among ED physicians, hospitalists, primary care physicians, and patients' families can prevent the discharge process from breaking down.

DIFFERENT TACTICS FOR DIFFERENT TYPES OF HOSPITALS

Readmission prevention tactics will depend on the setting and type of hospital. The following sections look at readmission prevention tactics specific to different types of hospitals. Some tactics will be more effective than others for each hospital type.

Rural Hospitals

Rural hospitals share certain characteristics that should be considered when developing a readmission plan. One of the most relevant data points that CMS shares with hospitals annually is the same-hospital readmission rate. A hospital with a same-hospital readmission rate lower than 60 percent is at risk for a readmission penalty because more than half of the patients return to another hospital. If this is the case at your hospital, then emphasizing patient education and access is critical. Same-hospital rates are even more relevant for rural hospitals because there are fewer hospitals in rural areas, and tracking your own readmission data is the biggest indicator of an overall problem. Rural hospitals often do not communicate with other hospitals in neighboring areas, and there may not be the consistent relationship and communication between hospitals that one often finds in metropolitan areas.

A rural setting provides an increased opportunity for collaboration between the acute care hospital and post-acute care providers because often there is only a small number of providers. Such opportunities range from the hospital's providing SNFs with clinical support and education to a coordinated community transition program. Many rural communities have already proven that these programs can be successful with the appropriate stakeholders.

Urban Settings

Access and convenience most often drive healthcare decisions in an urban setting. For example, patients often seek healthcare after they get home from work for the day, and they go to the ED because they assume they do not have any other choice after hours. Yet most metropolitan areas now offer several different access points to care after hours, and many health systems have teamed up with physicians to ensure that patients have access to physicians after hours. This has required creative solutions, and physicians who were historically competitive are now learning to work together.

Urban areas often present additional challenges to the same-hospital readmission rate. For example, when I was CEO of Western Medical Center Anaheim, a 188-bed acute care hospital near Disneyland, five competing acute care hospitals were located within five miles of our campus. Educating patients to always return to the same hospital was not likely to be effective, so other solutions needed to be considered, in particular connecting healthcare providers via the HIE. Connecting a community via the HIE requires acute care hospitals that have traditionally competed to share data through the HIE. Though it may take several months of planning, a truly connected community benefits the patients and the hospitals.

Urban hospitals have access to extensive community resources, and any hospital or health system that does not thoroughly investigate all available community resources is limiting itself. An organization that has extensive community resources at its disposal can capitalize on them to reduce costs and sometimes even get reimbursement while preventing readmissions.

Health Systems

Identifying specific tactics that a health system should implement to reduce readmissions is difficult because each health system is unique. However, the one tactic all health systems should consider is creating an HIE that is accessible by all providers and facilities in the network.

For health systems that have multiple hospitals in the same metropolitan area, many of these tactics can be implemented from one hospital to the next, regardless of which hospital the patient visited for the index stay. A true population management strategy would have similar or identical admitting criteria in each hospital and ED, and the focus would extend well beyond simple readmission prevention to include population health management.

For health systems that have hospitals spread out throughout the country, in urban areas or in both rural and urban areas, creating a system-wide approach would be wise to allow connectivity and create an alert system when patients are readmission candidates.

Academic and Teaching Hospitals

A unique characteristic of academic and teaching hospitals is that they usually have access to additional research dollars or grants that can help drive innovation in the areas of population health management and readmission prevention. Although the tactics to prevent readmissions in this setting are largely the same as in other hospitals, these additional resources and tools can be used to identify and study patients who are readmitted to the hospital unnecessarily.

Safety-Net or County Hospitals

I spent seven years operating safety-net hospitals as a CEO and took great pride in caring for underserved populations. In these safety-net hospitals I had no budget to address population management or readmission prevention—and on many days I had no operating cash in the bank. Yet even with such challenges, it is important to look beyond mere survival and identify effective readmission prevention tactics.

For example, an automated telephone system that calls high-risk patients after discharge is an effective tool for a safety-net hospital with a small budget. Several vendors offer this technology for a modest monthly fee, including Cipher Health, one of the leaders in this area. The patient is required to answer three questions by pressing a number on the phone. Questions are simple, such as, "Are you feeling better or worse than you did yesterday? Press one for better, two for the same, or three for worse."

Most hospital executives assume there would be a low response rate to this technology, but the opposite is the case when case managers and social workers educate patients before discharge to expect this call and emphasize the importance of taking two minutes to answer the questions. If the patient does not answer any of the questions, an alert is triggered to the hospital ambulatory case manager, and high-risk patient protocols are put into action.

Critical Access Hospitals

Although critical access hospitals are not subject to readmission penalties, they would still be wise to connect electronically with high-volume hospitals in the same region. Then, when a patient is admitted to a critical access hospital, the nurses and physicians would have access to the patient's medical history and be better prepared to address the patient's needs. In the post-ACA environment, healthcare providers at all levels should continue to move toward an integrated HIE so that the patient's medical history and genetic map can be referenced in his best interest.

SUMMARY

Regardless of the type of hospital, the future of healthcare is patient-centered care delivered in a value-based model. Creating a model where hospital admission is a last resort, reserved only for those who truly need acute care, takes two key commitments from providers. First, development of a comprehensive HIE allows providers at all levels to share as much data as possible about the patient (with the patient's consent). Second, physicians and hospitals alike must commit to using inpatient admission criteria that rule out all other options and are not financially motivated.

When health systems can commit to a minimum of two of the initiatives described in this chapter—sharing data and admitting patients only when truly necessary—the US healthcare system will finally reflect the model the ACA set out to create. Although progress is slow, the goal remains for healthcare organizations to convert from a fee-for-service model to a value-based model.

PERSPECTIVE
A Hospitalist's Perspective on Readmission Prevention

By Hassan Alkhouli, MD
Chief medical officer, Garden Grove (California) Medical Center

According to the Centers for Medicare & Medicaid Services (CMS), about 20 percent of Medicare patients are readmitted within 30 days of discharge from a hospital, most typically within the first 7 or 8 days of discharge (Jencks, Williams, and Coleman 2009). CMS also reports that half of these patients do not see a primary care physician for follow-up after their discharge. In 2004, unplanned readmissions cost Medicare approximately $17 billion, and the cost for potentially preventable readmissions was $12 billion. As many as 90 percent of these Medicare readmissions were unplanned.

Unplanned rehospitalizations for some of the most common diagnoses (e.g., heart failure, septicemia, simple pneumonia, dehydration, renal failure) are almost always critical emergencies, and although the patient's comorbid conditions play a role in readmission causes, most cases are the result of systems failures in ensuring appropriate transition to another source of care. Patients who are older than 80 years and have a history of depression, end-stage renal disease, or five or more chronic conditions pose the greatest risk for readmission, but that risk can be mitigated by recognizing their risk score early and tailoring a discharge plan that is most appropriate for their condition, including hospice and palliative care.

The primary contributor to the high readmission rate, however, is the breakdown of the discharge process. Historically, many patients who are readmitted to the hospital do not see their primary care physician within 7 to 14 days of discharge as recommended (American

→

Hospital Association and Health Research and Educational Trust 2014), even though many of them require additional outpatient workup. Often, discharge summaries are not readily available to primary care providers at the time of the postdischarge appointment, and even when the discharge summaries are accessible, most lack an accurate description of the hospital course of events, discharge medications, or any pending tests that may need further investigation. Patients are often not educated about the purpose of the drugs they are prescribed or about potential side effects. As a result, patients may not know the warning signs that could alert them to seek early medical advice.

Information technology–based improvements may help reduce rehospitalizations. Discharge summaries generated from the hospital database may include such important information as the physical exam, test results, pending results, and medications. Use of a discharge planner may also decrease readmission rates and, potentially, mortality rates.

Preventing readmissions is a challenging task because many internal and external factors contribute to the problem. However, improvement is possible with the implementation of changes in four areas:

1. *Communication among members of the care team:* Communication among the team members, including the hospital, primary care physician, specialist, patient, and transitional care specialist, can be anything from a simple phone call to an e-mail or a fax after the patient's discharge—when clear communication is key. The Society of Hospital Medicine (www.hospitalmedicine.org) has developed a discharge checklist that can be used to identify elements to include in a discharge summary and information

→

that needs to be communicated to the primary care physician after the patient becomes an outpatient.

2. *Medication reconciliation:* Reconciliation ensures that an accurate, up-to-date list of medications is maintained and is consistent with the patient's care plan. Regulatory agencies require this reconciliation to occur at discharge. The inpatient team needs to develop a standardized approach for reconciliation and education, whether provided by a physician or a nurse. The process can also be automated or involve the use of clinical pharmacists. Involving clinical pharmacists in the medication reconciliation process at discharge can lead to fewer adverse drug events after discharge and can reduce readmissions. In many of the more robust pharmacist-based programs, patients are called after discharge to troubleshoot medication problems.

3. *Pending tests and labs:* Many patients are discharged with laboratory and other test results pending. Physicians are often unaware of tests requiring review and follow-up after hospital discharge. Although automated mechanisms to track pending results are the ideal, they remain uncommon. Creating checklists and extra layers of safety for important results (i.e., having more than one follow-up appointment scheduled with the care provider) and communicating what action should be taken in response to the pending test result will help ensure that important results are not overlooked.

4. *Patient- and family-empowerment discharge coaches:* Involving the patient or family in the discharge process has been associated with improved outcomes by providing an extra layer of safety for follow-up of test results pending at discharge and communicating important events that occurred during the

$\longrightarrow$

hospitalization. Encouraging patients to take a more active role in their care and providing tools and guidance in the form of transition coaches can lower hospital costs and readmission rates for elderly patients. This patient-centered approach is a useful strategy to improve care transitions.

In conclusion, communication should not be restricted to simply the doctor–patient relationship but should encompass the relationships between the emergency department physician and hospitalist, the hospitalist and the primary care physician, and the primary care physician and the family. Proper documents, including laboratory and diagnostic test results and discharge summaries, should be readily available to all care providers. The healthcare community at large can also play a role in making transitional care more efficient among the local population. Partnerships may be built between hospitals and other healthcare providers and community agencies to facilitate easy access to patient documents, allowing direct lines of communication between facilities and supplying healthcare providers with critical information regarding their patient population.

REFERENCES

American Hospital Association and Health Research and Educational Trust. 2014. *Improving Care Transitions and Reducing Readmissions: 2014 Update.* Chicago: AHA/HRET.

Jencks, S. F., M. V. Williams, and E. A. Coleman. 2009. "Rehospitalizations Among Patients in the Medicare Fee-for-Service Program." *New England Journal of Medicine* 360 (14): 1418–28.

CHAPTER 8

Readmission Prevention for Post-Acute Care Providers

If you have worked in the post-acute care sector, then you know that quality, differentiation, and accessibility are the key drivers that position a post-acute care facility or agency to succeed. The fee-for-service reimbursement model created a financially lucrative opportunity for post-acute care providers and led to significant growth in the sector over the past 20 years. The crowding in the post-acute care space is evident from the many post-acute care providers trying to plead their case with the hospital case management department as to why their agency or facility is better than the others and should be the provider of choice.

At times the crowding has led to unprofessional marketing practices between post-acute care providers and their hospital referral sources, and regulatory lines have sometimes been crossed. Post-acute care marketers have traditionally given food, gifts, and other inducements to discharge planners and case managers to win their favor and gain their business. Although this practice is still common, regulatory agencies and hospital owners have increased their scrutiny and tightened their policies on such marketing tactics, with the result that a lot of the inducements have gone away or been scaled back to reasonably priced items. To ensure a consistent flow of referrals, post-acute care providers have had to change their approach and become more skilled at marketing the unique characteristics that set them apart from their competition. The result has been innovative thinking, new specialty programs, improved customer service, and quicker response times once the referral is received.

PRIOR APPROACH TO REFERRALS

In the 1990s and the first decade of the new millennium, the goal of a post-acute provider was to become a preferred provider of therapy services in the skilled-nursing sector. Medicare only pays for skilled days in a nursing home, and skilled days translate to therapy days, so the name of the game was becoming the best-known therapy provider in your area.

Skilled-nursing facilities (SNFs) that could ensure quality outcomes, aggressive therapy, the patient's safe return home, and a high level of patient satisfaction on discharge were likely to become the provider of choice for hospital case managers and discharge planners. Once the word was out that a certain SNF was the leader in therapy service delivery and patient satisfaction, the word would spread to primary care physicians, hospitalists, health plans, and managed care organizations and that facility would start to see significant volume growth and success.

Many SNFs allocated substantial resources to differentiate their facilities and position themselves as superior to other SNFs. The facilities' CEOs, chief nursing officers, marketing liaisons, and nurse liaisons all received extensive training to equip them to market their strengths to hospital case managers. Post-acute care marketers and liaisons were even known to study a hospital's security and discharge planning structure to determine the best way to gain access to patients, physicians, and discharge planners.

Similarly, home health agencies and hospice organizations that provided a high level of service and had strong customer satisfaction became the providers of choice for hospitals and preferred SNF providers. In many cases, hospital discharge planners took advantage of the antisteering inpatient choice laws put in place by the Centers for Medicare & Medicaid Services to protect a patient's choice and steered patients to their preferred facility. This is not to suggest that they did so with ill intentions. Though there were inappropriate referrals in this era, discharge planners often steered patients in the direction of preferred providers because their quality and patient satisfaction were consistently strong.

TODAY'S APPROACH TO REFERRALS

The key selling point in the post-acute care sector—both then and now—is quality. Quality outcomes, quick referral response times, differentiation, and customer satisfaction have always driven the leading SNFs, but today there is a new priority: a low facility readmission rate.

After the Affordable Care Act (ACA) was signed into law in 2010, post-acute care providers turned their focus to readmission prevention as a key differentiator. However, most post-acute care providers had no idea how to operationalize readmission prevention or document it to show hospitals that they were aggressively preventing readmissions. As a result, there was a lot of talk in the post-acute care space about working hard to prevent readmissions but few models and case studies emerged to demonstrate actual strategic planning or efforts to collaborate with hospitals to prevent readmissions.

The amount of turnover at SNFs and other post-acute care agencies is notably higher than in other healthcare sectors, and creating and implementing a strategic plan from start to finish can be difficult because the personalities and leadership often change midstream. One of the biggest challenges in the population management era is that acute care hospital leaders have little knowledge about the inner workings of the different levels of post-acute care. The post-acute care sector, in turn, has little knowledge about acute care operations. The primary difference, however, is that although post-acute care leaders have been studying the acute care model for more than 30 years, they still struggle to find ways to get the attention and focus of acute care leaders. Until the ACA passed, acute care leaders seemed not to care. Only a few acute care organizations have started to engage the post-acute care community in adapting to a population management model, but by the end of 2016 more than half of the hospitals nationwide will likely have engaged local post-acute care providers in some way, whether formally or informally.

CHALLENGES FACING THE HEALTHCARE INDUSTRY

The dilemma facing the healthcare industry today is that although the ACA has been a reality for several years, most of the acute care sector resists adapting to a value-based reimbursement model. Yet adaptation is essential to future viability. Independent hospitals will not be able to survive as stand-alone businesses—for-profit hospitals in particular, but not-for-profit hospitals as well. Unless a hospital is part of a health system that has innovative leaders who are looking for new and nontraditional revenue streams, the hospital is unlikely to be able to generate enough revenue to operate and provide inpatient services in the future, particularly with added risk factors such as high overhead, significant inpatient infrastructure, and high wages for unionized inpatient nurses and aides.

Whether the health system is creating new revenue streams by starting wellness and healthy lifestyle ventures, leasing out space in the hospital or community, operating a hospital coffee shop or restaurant, or launching nontraditional service lines (e.g., assisted living, freestanding skilled nursing, home health, home care, hospice), hospitals must start to make up for the impending loss of inpatient revenue as soon as possible. Hospitals still have significant influence in the healthcare space, but as that influence wanes in coming years, starting new business ventures will become more difficult for them.

Your hospital's chief financial officer should project how the future healthcare model will affect your facility by creating a pro forma budget using the existing cost structure but reducing the current inpatient revenue by 40 percent (because a 30 percent decrease in inpatient admissions is likely by the end of 2015). Once that exercise is complete, look at the new bottom line and discuss the hospital's continued viability if that reduction in revenue becomes a reality.

The next step is to start identifying new revenue streams that can compensate for at least a portion of the lost revenue. Although the new revenue streams will probably not make up for the full 40 percent loss in revenue, the only alternative is reducing overhead and staff. New revenue streams, such as home health services and healthy lifestyle gymnasiums, however small, are a good approach to start chipping away at the projected loss.

The other reason to start thinking about how to generate new revenue as soon as possible, whether in traditional or nontraditional hospital business models, is so that you can retain as much of your current staff as possible. However, some reduction in the number of full-time staff needed for the delivery of inpatient services is a certainty: It has already happened at many historically successful hospitals and health systems and will continue to happen to the point that some hospitals will not be able to continue to operate, resulting in hospital consolidation, acquisition, or closure. The end result will be the rich getting richer and the poor going away as the bigger and more lucrative health systems swallow up the facilities worth keeping open and the others shut down.

WHERE DOES THE READMISSIONS ISSUE FIT?

Although readmission penalties are coming to SNFs in 2017—and likely to other post-acute care levels in the future—the key motivating factor for post-acute care operators will not be their own readmission penalty but staying in the good graces of the hospital that feeds them. Post-acute care providers cannot operate without referrals from their high-volume acute care partners. They must keep the referrals flowing. Beyond providing quality care, referrals will always be the top priority for post-acute care providers.

In summary, although many acute care operators have still not prioritized readmissions as a relevant topic in their boardrooms, post-acute care providers must continue to showcase their commitment to readmission prevention and their success in preventing unnecessary hospital readmissions to their key referral sources. Post-acute care providers have a captive audience in hospital case managers and discharge planners who are advocates for their patients. Case managers want to work with post-acute care providers who are committed to preventing unnecessary readmissions.

Therefore, post-acute care providers must prioritize, strategize, communicate, and track readmissions. Post-acute care providers who are not prioritizing readmissions and using the tactics described in this book should not expect to be in existence five years from now because the ACA has laid the groundwork for hospitals to narrow their network and work only with those providers that are committed to maintaining high quality and preventing unnecessary readmissions.

CHAPTER 9

Preventing Readmissions in Skilled-Nursing Facilities

Although many hospital administrators have hesitated to engage post-acute care providers in readmission prevention and other population-management strategies, skilled-nursing facilities (SNFs) must make readmission prevention a top priority. Beyond delivering quality outcomes, ensuring patient satisfaction, and running a profitable operation, preventing unnecessary hospital readmissions should be an SNF administrator's top priority because it is the means by which a facility sets itself apart from the others.

Quality will always be the first requirement when a hospital makes a referral to a post-acute care provider, but an SNF must succeed in several key areas to be considered a preferred provider:

- Quality
- Patient satisfaction
- Accessibility (i.e., open beds should consistently be available)
- Ease of referral/discharge process
- Response to referral times

And now, in the post–Affordable Care Act (ACA) era, one more key area should be added:

- Readmission prevention

With this in mind, an administrator's challenge in developing a readmission prevention strategy for his SNF is making sure staff are trained to handle and care for as many clinical needs and situations as possible. An administrator's top priority in readmission prevention can be summed up as follows:

The SNF is responsible for preventing the patient from leaving the facility to return to a hospital.

In short, keep the patient in your facility whenever possible. Hospitals are not measuring SNFs so much on their readmission rate as on their competency in caring for patients and not sending them to the emergency department (ED) unnecessarily. Thus, nursing home administrators should focus on the return-to-ED rate, not the return-to-acute-care rate. Once a patient is in the ED, the SNF has no control over readmission because the hospital makes the readmission decision. Thus, the SNF administrator should manage the situation at her end by being aware of every patient in her facility who leaves for any reason to go to any hospital. When the administrator makes this a priority, discusses all return-to-ED patients every morning at her facility's stand-up meeting, and shows a consistent commitment to preventing unnecessary readmissions, facility culture will follow.

To help prevent patients from having to leave the SNF, tools such as the INTERACT (Interventions to Reduce Acute Care Transfers) protocols are invaluable because they give step-by-step directions for nurses to follow when a patient's state declines. In the fee-for-service model, when a patient started to decline an SNF nurse would tell the physician, and the physician's response was to send the patient to the ED. This response was not only convenient for the physician but was also the safest approach.

Under the fee-for-service model, a physician was reimbursed each time a patient went to the hospital, and the hospital was reimbursed each time a patient came to its ED—and again if he was admitted to the hospital. Under the fee-for-service model, the

SNF required a patient to spend three midnights in a hospital for her Medicare benefit to cover therapy services once she returned to the SNF. Often, when a patient was declining, she had been in the SNF for several months, was no longer receiving therapy services, and was considered a long-term resident receiving custodial care. Thus, by returning to the hospital and staying three midnights, the patient could return to the SNF eligible to be covered for therapy services by Medicare.

Traditionally, reimbursement for custodial or long-term care in an SNF ranged from $120 to $190 per day. By comparison, diagnosis-related group (DRG) reimbursement for Medicare patients receiving therapy services usually ranges from $300 to $750 per day. This is why Medicare is king in SNFs and facilities are always improving and showcasing their therapy services as a key differentiator. Therapy, skilled days (length of stay), and the Medicare benefit are the key drivers of financial success at an SNF.

Although the average length of stay for a therapy patient in an SNF traditionally ranges between 14 and 20 days, over the past 20 years owners and operators have become skilled at justifying extended lengths of stay. In some facilities, the average length of stay was more than 30 days. Although extended lengths of stay were tough to justify in any environment, they are an example of how operators who studied the DRG system, therapy services, and reimbursement were able to maximize their revenues and at the same time ensure quality outcomes.

In a post-ACA environment, SNF length of stay is already coming under scrutiny. Just as hospital operators are struggling to adapt to population management and value-based reimbursement models, SNF administrators are coming to grips with the fact that they will need to shorten lengths of stay, which is contradictory to everything they have been trained to do. The danger here is that the administrators may tell the hospital and health plan whatever they want to hear to get the contract or business. Under a post-ACA model, competing interests related to length of stay will persist between the staff and the payer for a long time to come. Longer SNF stays reflect poorly on the referring hospital and the SNF because commercial payers are always seeking to reduce costs and because new programs continue to be added annually to the ACA that penalize hospitals if their post-acute care providers have higher-than-expected utilization and costs. Unless you find a system that is highly integrated in a community committed to coordinated care or an integrated network with a vibrant accountable care organization (ACO), bundled-payment program, or lucrative risk-sharing arrangement that includes the SNF, the SNF will almost certainly retain a mindset to extend length of stay for Medicare and managed care patients who are receiving therapy. The sooner an administrator can discard this way of thinking, the likelier his SNF will be included in ACOs, bundled-payment programs, and risk-sharing arrangements.

Following are readmission prevention tactics that build on those introduced in Part II, along with a brief description of how they should be applied in a skilled-nursing setting.

MAKE SURE POLST FORMS ARE AVAILABLE FOR ALL PATIENTS

Skilled-nursing leadership must make sure that every patient has a Physician Orders for Life-Sustaining Treatment (POLST) form in his chart at the nursing station. A copy of the POLST form should also be placed in a plastic sleeve and hung on or near the door in the patient's room so that if 911 emergency services are called or the patient is transported to the hospital, the paramedics can grab the plastic sleeve and take the POLST form with them to the hospital.

Nurses should always send a copy of the POLST form when the patient transfers to the hospital. For this reason, three copies of the POLST form should be inside the chart at all times because the hospital rarely sends it back when the patient returns to the SNF.

Most SNFs will claim they use the POLST form for all patients. However, a check of patient charts at the nursing station often shows that the POLST forms are not there. The nursing home administrator and the director of nursing should be equally committed to enforcing the practice of having three copies of the POLST form in all patient charts at all times. When this commitment is made and demonstrated at the top, it becomes part of the facility's culture and makes the facility stand out to referral partners.

CONDUCT OR GAIN ACCESS TO PATIENT RISK ASSESSMENTS

The SNF is not necessarily responsible for performing patient risk stratifications, but caretakers at all levels must understand which patients are at high risk for readmission. The hospital and health system likely have significant resources and expensive tools to perform risk assessments, so the SNF's goal is to gain access to these risk tools to make sure the SNF and its caretakers are aware of high-risk patients when they arrive. Additionally, SNFs should have a protocol for high-risk patients—at a minimum, to raise awareness that the patient is a "frequent flyer" at the hospital. Although a variety of protocols are available to identify high-risk patients, the important point is that the SNF must have a protocol and the SNF's leaders must communicate its importance. When staff leaders make identifying high-risk patients a priority, staff will follow their example.

PARTICIPATE IN POST-ACUTE CARE NETWORKS AND COMMUNITY COLLABORATIVES

All SNF administrators should seek out post-acute care networks and community collaboratives in their area. The meeting topics are not nearly as important as your presence. When a facility does not show up to the meeting, it sends a message to the hospital that readmissions are not a priority and the hospital is not an important referral source.

If the hospitals that refer to you do not have their own post-acute care network and there is no community collaborative, consider taking the lead in forming a community collaborative using one of these strategies:

- If multiple hospitals refer to your facility, offer to host a community collaborative meeting and let the facilities attending the meeting dictate the agenda.
- If there is only one hospital referral source in your area, offer to organize a meeting but encourage participants to refer to it as the hospital's post-acute care network rather than your post-acute care network. Connecting your facility to the hospital serves as an indirect endorsement of your facility. As the hospital's case management team and leadership become more aware of your SNF, you will become even more of a preferred provider and receive more referrals.

MAKE SURE YOU ARE PART OF THE HOSPITAL'S NARROW NETWORK

SNFs must lobby to be included in any narrow network. Hospitals are narrowing their networks—rather than referring to all the SNFs in their region, they may refer to only a few preferred providers. Although this practice seems antithetical to patient choice and anti-steering regulations, the ACA incentivizes hospitals to narrow their network and penalizes them if they do not. Patient choice and anti-steering regulations remain in place, but hospitals have found creative ways to steer patients to their post-acute care facilities and providers of choice while still allowing patients to believe they had a choice.

Administrators should not waste time worrying about whether it is legal or appropriate if a hospital takes such action. Instead, spend your energy making sure your SNF is one of the preferred providers in the narrow network. If your SNF is not initially included in the hospital's narrow network, do not give up. Continue to deliver data monthly, regularly communicate with and market to the hospital, reach out to the C-suite to state your case, and engage physicians who are loyal to your facility and active at the hospital. In short, use any method you can to be included. The reality is that patients can still choose your facility.

Be sure to examine your marketing strategies. I have noted that post-acute care providers often have inconsistent marketing approaches—aggressive for a month or two and then nonexistent for a month or two. I recommend that post-acute care providers deliver data to the hospital on the fifteenth of each month, including readmission statistics, patient DNA maps (see Exhibit 9.1 for an example), and any other information that would set the facility apart from the rest. Before long, the hospital will expect your data to show up mid-month.

Also, understand what weaknesses could prevent your facility from being included in a narrow network. Consider proximity, for example. Is your facility in a hospital's 911 zone, or are you closer to another hospital? Proximity is often the top factor a hospital considers when deciding whether to include you in its narrow network. Hospitals do not want to send their patients to a facility in an area where the paramedics would be required to take 911 patients to another hospital. Do not underestimate proximity as a deciding factor for hospitals.

Administrators should investigate county regulations regarding which hospital paramedics are required to take patients to. In most counties, paramedics are encouraged to take the patient back to the hospital he came from and honor patient choice, but in an advanced cardiac life support or other emergency situation, paramedics are usually required to go to the nearest ED. Once you understand

Exhibit 9.1 Sample Genetics Report

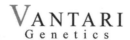

Genetic Technological Innovations, LLC • 15440 Laguna Canyon Road, • Suite 260 • Irvine, CA 92618 • P: 949.783.5300 • F: 949.783.5302
Laboratory Director: Mario Kohan, MD

Vantari Panel Report Created for: Joe Vantari test

Patient:	Joe Vantari test		DOB:	9/5/1976
Accession #:	#875		Gender:	
Collection Date:			Received Date:	
Ordered By:	Dr Bowe		Report Generated:	2/3/2014

Test Details

Gene	Genotype	Phenotype
CYP2C19	*17/*17	Rapid Metabolizer
CYP2C9	*1/*3	Intermediate Metabolizer
CYP2D6	*3/*3	Poor Metabolizer
CYP3A4	*1/*1	Normal Metabolizer
CYP3A5	*1/*3	Intermediate Metabolizer
Factor II	20210G>A GG	Normal Thrombosis Risk
Factor V Leiden	1691G>A AA	High Thrombosis Risk
MTHFR	1298A>C AA	No Increased Risk of Hyperhomocysteinemia
MTHFR	677C>T TT	Increased Risk of Hyperhomocysteinemia
VKORC1	-1639G>A G/G	Low Warfarin Sensitivity

Disclaimer

The information presented on this report is provided as general educational health information. The Content is not intended to be a substitute for professional medical advice, diagnosis, or treatment. Only a physician, pharmacist or other healthcare professional should advise a patient on the use of the medications prescribed.

Patient Medications

Current Medication List: Trazodone, Amitriptyline, Oxymorphone, Phenytoin

Medications Affected by Patient Genetic Results

Amitriptyline (Elavil)

Increased Sensitivity to Amitriptyline (CYP2C19 *17/*17 Rapid Metabolizer)

Consider an alternative drug or consider prescribing amitriptyline at standard dose and monitor the plasma concentrations of amitriptyline and nortriptyline to guide dose adjustments.

Phenytoin (Dilantin)

Moderate Sensitivity to Phenytoin (CYP2C9 *1/*3 Intermediate Metabolizer)

Consider a standard loading dose and reduce maintenance dose by 25%. Evaluate response and serum concentrations after 7-10 days. Be alert to neurological concentration-related adverse events.

Patient Medications for which there is no clinically established Pharmacogenetic Guidance*:

Trazodone, Oxymorphone

* Medications that are metabolized by multiple enzymes, or by enzymes which activity varies very little among individuals are expected to be less sensitive to the pharmacogenetic markers detected by this assay.

Genetic Test Results For Joe Vantari test

(continued)

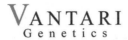

Genetic Technological Innovations, LLC • 15440 Laguna Canyon Road, • Suite 260 • Irvine, CA 92618 • P: 949.783.5300 • F: 949.783.5302
Laboratory Director: Mario Kohan, MD

Potentially Impacted Medications

	Cardiovascular Medications
⚑	Metoprolol (Lopressor)
⚠	Carvedilol (Coreg), Clopidogrel (Plavix), Flecainide (Tambocor), Fluvastatin (Lescol), Mexiletine (Mexitil), Propafenone (Rythmol), Timolol (Timoptic), Warfarin (Coumadin)
✓	Irbesartan (Avapro), Nebivolol (Bystolic), Prasugrel (Effient), Propranolol (Inderal), Ticagrelor (Brilinta)

	Pain Medications
⚑	Codeine (Codeine), Tramadol (Ultram)
⚠	Carisoprodol (Soma), Celecoxib (Celebrex)
✓	Flurbiprofen (Ansaid), Hydrocodone (Vicodin), Oxycodone (Percocet), Piroxicam (Feldene)

	Psychotropic Medications
⚑	Amitriptyline (Elavil), Citalopram (Celexa), Clomipramine (Anafranil), Desipramine (Norpramin), Doxepin (Silenor), Escitalopram (Lexapro), Haloperidol (Haldol), Imipramine (Tofranil), Nortriptyline (Pamelor), Risperidone (Risperdal), Thioridazine (Mellaril), Trimipramine (Surmontil), Venlafaxine (Effexor)
⚠	Aripiprazole (Abilify), Atomoxetine (Strattera), Diazepam (Valium), Donepezil (Aricept), Duloxetine (Cymbalta), Galantamine (Razadyne), Iloperidone (Fanapt), Paroxetine (Paxil), Perphenazine (Trilafon), Phenytoin (Dilantin), Pimozide (Orap), Tetrabenazine (Xenazine)
✓	Clobazam (Onfi), Clozapine (Clozaril), Desvenlafaxine (Pristiq), Mirtazapine (Remeron), Olanzapine (Zyprexa), Paliperidone (Invega), Sertraline (Zoloft)

	Other Medications
⚑	None
⚠	Darifenacin (Enablex), Dexlansoprazole (Dexilant), Esomeprazole (Nexium), Lansoprazole (Prevacid), Omeprazole (Prilosec), Pantoprazole (Protonix), Tacrolimus (Prograf), Tamsulosin (Flomax), Tolterodine (Detrol), Voriconazole (Vfend)
✓	Fesoterodine (Toviaz), Glimepiride (Amaryl), Glipizide (Glucotrol), Glyburide (Micronase), Ondansetron (Zofran), Rabeprazole (Aciphex), Tolbutamide (Orinase)

Source: Vantari Genetics, LLC. Used with permission.

Chapter 9: Preventing Readmissions in Skilled-Nursing Facilities   147 local regulations, you can start to understand the politics that drive paramedic routes. For example, find out where their base station is. After they drop off a patient and are between calls, paramedics are often required to park at one of the major hospitals in the area. They will always be subconsciously incentivized to take patients to that hospital because it will maximize their time and convenience. Other factors that influence paramedics' decisions and willingness to divert patients to an ED other than the one they are supposed to include hospitals providing free meals or snacks and the desire to see a friend or spouse who works at the hospital.

All of these factors are still relevant if it is the health plan or insurer that is narrowing the network. Understand the goals of the narrow network and who is driving it, and work relentlessly to be included.

IDENTIFY LOCAL TRANSITIONAL CARE PROGRAMS

SNF administrators should first identify which transitional care program is being used by the hospital or in the community, then read up on the specific program and make sure employees are prepared to fulfill their role in the process.

For example, several transitional care programs require a post-acute care follow-up visit to a primary care physician or high-risk patient clinic. Some hospitals ask the SNF to schedule that appointment after discharge from the SNF. Nursing homes are under no obligation to do so, but complying with the request is one way to stay in the hospital's good graces.

The SNF may also consider pushing the hospital to connect with the SNF electronically, creating a true community health information exchange (HIE). Because the hospital will likely not make this a priority, the SNF must advocate for a community HIE with the hospital's influential physicians.

PROVIDE AMBULATORY CASE MANAGEMENT SERVICES

Ambulatory case management refers to monitoring, servicing, and assisting the patient beyond discharge from the hospital to an SNF. One of the benefits of narrowing the home health network is that it can manage the process on behalf of the hospital and SNF.

However, when a patient discharged from the SNF to home is not enrolled in a home health network, many hospitals look to the SNF to provide a follow-up visit or place a phone call to the patient. SNFs that undertake home visits for their discharged patients are rare, so if a facility has the resources to provide this service consistently, this key differentiator would position the facility as a preferred provider with the referring hospital. At a minimum, however, the SNF should place a follow-up call within 72 hours and another at the end of the first week after discharge.

The main goals of the phone calls or visit are to

- confirm that the patient has safely transferred to her living environment,
- ensure that the patient understands her medication regimen and has an adequate supply of medication,
- ensure that the patient is comfortable and not anxious about self-management or her living environment, and
- identify risk factors visually on a home visit or through questions on a phone call.

Following are the four main questions asked on follow-up phone calls:

1. Are you feeling better or worse than the day you were discharged from the facility?
2. Do you have any questions about your medication?

3. Do you have an adequate supply of all of your medications?
4. Do you have any other questions or concerns that are making you anxious about your recovery care at home?

Note that the first three questions require a yes or no answer, whereas the fourth question is open ended and gives the patient an opportunity to share any anxieties about the discharge. The call should not be made on the day of discharge, and if the practice is to place the call within 24 hours of discharge, the evening of the day after discharge is best. Any time a patient in the recovery process is transferred from one location to another, fatigue, pain, anxiety about the unknown, and other factors come into play. Calling 48 to 72 hours after discharge is recommended because the goal is to identify concerns and adverse conditions beyond the transfer process and to see if there are any roadblocks now that the patient has returned to his living environment.

PROVIDE REMOTE MONITORING SERVICES

A great way for an SNF to set itself apart from its competition is to partner with a hospital and physician to operate a remote monitoring unit. In many states, Medicare is now reimbursing for remote monitoring devices. On discharge from the hospital, physicians can prescribe one of many different monitoring devices that will shorten hospital length of stay and allow a patient to return home from the hospital sooner.

Many physicians have found that an even better solution can be discharging the patient to an SNF that operates a remote monitoring unit with specially trained nurses. The investment for an SNF to open such a unit is minimal.

The remote monitoring process is simple. The remote device is applied to the patient in the hospital or the physician's office and remains in place while the patient is a resident at the SNF. The patient's vital signs are relayed via wireless technology to a data center that knows the patient's location and has a direct telephone number to the SNF nursing desk. If a patient's remote monitoring device alerts the command center of a change in vital signs, the data center immediately notifies the SNF about the changing condition.

Remote monitoring is popular in cardiac care. To start a cardiac remote monitoring unit, the SNF needs the following:

- *A program director:* Finding a cardiologist to champion the effort may be the most difficult step. Consider setting aside a modest stipend for a cardiologist to oversee the program, monitor quality, and recommend improvements to better care for cardiac patients who are being monitored remotely. These responsibilities can often be difficult in an SNF environment because cardiologists may not consider a modest stipend to be enough to justify their spending time at an SNF.
- *A unit or wing in the facility:* To find an appropriate location for the cardiac remote monitoring unit, start by identifying the corridors that can be created by closing existing doors in the hallway (possibly fire corridor doors). A cardiac remote monitoring unit is not likely to have a high volume of patients, so any corridor with 12 or fewer beds would be an ideal location. To maximize efficiencies and bed capacity, the SNF should consider expanding the unit to include remote monitoring patients with conditions other than cardiac problems.
- *Signage and unit naming:* Once a cardiologist and an area of the facility are identified, the SNF should post signage to brand the service area and direct visitors. Many facilities place a framed picture of the unit director next to the name of the unit, identifying her as the unit director of the cardiac remote monitoring unit or cardiac rehabilitation unit. Note that in some states you need to be careful if you call something a "unit" because the state department of health may have specific requirements for such entities.

- *Nurse training and competency:* An SNF can open a cardiac remote monitoring service with relative ease by identifying one physician who supports the initiative and is willing to apply the technology and bill Medicare. The facility's nursing staff need basic training on how the process works, specifically how to contact the command center and what steps to take if a patient's condition changes.

COLLECT FACILITY-SPECIFIC DATA

Knowledge is power. Know your SNF data, and know it as soon as possible because Centers for Medicare & Medicaid Services reports are often delayed by more than a year. Whether you partner with COMS Interactive, PointRight, Servarus, or another software provider, each has a quality report that includes readmission data and can be generated each month.

These data should be reviewed by your clinical staff and leadership team and should also be shared with your hospital partners. Exhibit 3.1 (in Chapter 3) is a sample COMS Interactive report that shows the type of data your team should be reviewing and sending to the hospital each month. Hospitals are interested in this information and may not have access to it themselves.

CONNECT VIA A HEALTH
INFORMATION EXCHANGE

All SNFs should be committed to connecting electronically with their key referral partners as soon as possible. Many hospitals and health systems have not yet reached out to post-acute care providers to connect via HIEs, but once the incentives and deadlines have passed for hospitals to implement electronic health records, hospitals will begin to look outward and realize the importance of connecting with their post-acute care providers.

Post-acute care providers should not wait for the hospital to engage them in this conversation, however—they should start researching the hospital's connectivity requirements and software providers so that when the hospital is ready to have the discussion, they are prepared to quickly integrate. Much discussion will be needed to make the connectivity a reality, but by the end of 2016 it will be more common for hospitals to be connected to post-acute care providers via an HIE.

HAVE A CONSISTENT MARKETING PLAN

Although SNFs market aggressively to referral partners, those efforts are often inconsistent. Creating a strategic and specific marketing plan can help SNFs reach out to referral partners consistently and effectively.

Providing data about your facility should be a critical component of your marketing efforts. Monthly data are typically not available until around the tenth of the following month, so on the fifteenth of each month the skilled-nursing marketer should deliver an information package to each of his key contacts at the hospital.

The information package should include monthly readmission reports, remote monitoring success stories, genetic test results and case summaries for each patient referred from that hospital in the prior month, and a handwritten note from the marketer thanking the contact for her business and noting that the marketer is available to answer any questions. The marketer should be sure to indicate that he will be back in touch on the fifteenth of the next month with new readmission data and genetic maps.

Hospitals do not always access their readmission data. Thus, an SNF that consistently delivers these data each month and provides the hospital with a well-prepared information package will set itself apart from the others as a preferred provider that is committed to coordinated and patient-centered care.

PROMOTE SELF-MANAGEMENT, PATIENT HEALTH LITERACY, AND USE OF TEACH-BACK METHODS

Patient self-management is the most critical way to prevent readmissions at every level of care. Every administrator should make sure that staff—particularly the director of nursing, nurses, nurse aides, social workers, therapists, and discharge planners—are all committed to educating patients to care for themselves.

The ultimate goal is to get the patient home safely, and the post-acute care provider's challenge is to understand the patient's home environment. No matter what the home environment is like, however, all patients need to learn to care for themselves or else readmission is inevitable. Patient health literacy is necessary for effective self-management. In short, the patient must have a clear understanding of how to best care for his needs.

Teach-back is the methodology most commonly used to ensure patient health literacy. In this patient-education method, the patient is provided with collateral material illustrating what she has learned and is then asked to confirm comprehension by reciting back or demonstrating the protocols she needs to self-administer her care. The SNF should never underestimate its role in this process.

If the SNF hopes to be included in a narrow network and be viewed as a preferred provider, it must take an active, calculated role in fulfilling the educational mission of the transitional care program, post-acute care network, or community collaborative. Ignoring this piece of the process and assuming that the acute care hospital, health plan, or home health agency will ensure patient health literacy would be naive and short-sighted for an SNF.

PURSUE CONTRACT ALIGNMENT

Given the focus on preventing readmissions and the national trend toward absorbing Medicare patients into managed care, it is more critical than ever that SNFs have significant contract alignment. As the ACA has shifted the influence away from the hospital and physician in the coordinated care model, health plans and insurers have gained even more influence in the process. Thus, all SNFs should be aggressively seeking contracts and no longer relying on Medicare patients to cover the cost of operations. In fact, in states such as California, where all Medicare fee-for-service patients will likely be absorbed into managed care within the next five years, SNF operators would be wise to start planning and budgeting operations without Medicare patients. Instead, they should use a lower per diem and count traditional Medicare patients as managed care patients. Although many may consider this a doomsday approach, a facility that prepares itself in this manner will be successful regardless of how the delivery system evolves.

CONDUCT GENETIC TESTING

One of the most important technological medical advances in recent years is the availability of DNA testing and genetic mapping. SNFs have begun to see the value in ordering genetic tests to better manage patients' medication regimens, reduce medication errors, and lower overall medication costs to the SNF.

The procedure, which is covered by Medicare Part B as of January 1, 2014, may be conducted once in a patient's lifetime. The hospital community has been slow to order genetic maps because the benefit is not approved under Medicare Part A and because hospitals are not reimbursed for inpatients. Many SNFs, however, recognize that genetic testing not only is a means to improve patient care but also gives them a marketing advantage over their competition, and they have begun ordering these tests for their patients and sharing results with the referring hospital partner to be scanned into the patient's electronic health record for permanent use.

Many physicians have told me the technology is useful, is proven, and works. Many believe that within five years DNA tests will be standard for all newborns because the technology is so useful. A number of labs are currently conducting genetic testing. Exhibit 9.1 shows a sample report from Vantari Genetics in Irvine, California.

The most important thing for SNFs to understand about genetic testing is that it is in the best interest of the patient and will reduce the overall costs of providing care—outcomes that are consistent with the goals of the ACA. In addition, a commitment to genetic testing will distinguish a facility from its competition and mark it as an innovative partner in the coordinated care model. As noted elsewhere in this chapter, delivering genetic test results to the hospital is an effective marketing strategy. After obtaining the proper consent, the hospital will appreciate being able to scan the report and summary into the patient's electronic health record for use by everyone connected to the HIE.

NARROW THE HOME HEALTH NETWORK AND COORDINATE HOME HEALTH SERVICES

An SNF that is a true partner in a coordinated care model proactively ensures that the patient's discharge home is safe and that a fluid transition exists for continued rehabilitation and therapy services if needed. Although a patient may not always need home health services after discharge from an SNF, elderly patients should always be evaluated for home health services on discharge.

The ACA incentivizes providers to coordinate care to ensure a patient's well-being and avoid unnecessary hospital admissions. When a physician writes an order for home health services on discharge from any level of care, the order is for an evaluation. If the home health provider evaluates the patient in his home and determines that he is strong enough and well enough to care for himself in the absence of home health services, nothing is lost by having the evaluation done. Thus, all patients being discharged from an SNF should be given a physician's order for a home health evaluation.

Although the number of home health agencies increased significantly during the fee-for-service era, the ACA was a turning point and the number of agencies began to shrink. In an effort to best coordinate care, hospitals are using a hospital-owned home health agency, partnering with a single home health agency, or narrowing their network of home health agencies, sometimes to only three preferred providers.

One of the most critical factors for SNFs in this process is that they know which home health agencies are used by their key referring hospitals. In fact, if the SNF is acting in the best interest of the patient and the coordinated care model, it would consider eliminating all other home health agencies it refers to other than those used by the hospital from which the patient was transferred.

As a hypothetical example, if County Hospital has narrowed its network to Home Health A, Home Health B, and Home Health C, then the SNF should discharge patients transferred from the hospital only to one of these three home health agencies. If the SNF's leaders do not make a calculated and firm decision to implement this practice, the SNF is at risk of being dropped as a preferred provider by that hospital. Knowing that SNFs rely on hospital discharges to operate, leaders should be careful in choosing the home health agencies the SNF partners with.

INVEST IN PREDICTIVE SOFTWARE

SNFs that are committed to preventing readmissions and coordinating care with their referral partners invest in predictive software.

The software allows early identification of a patient who is declining, alerts the care team, and provides a pathway and recommendations on how best to stabilize the patient so that a hospital readmission is avoided.

Many facilities think they do not need to invest in software because they use INTERACT tools for the same purpose. However, there is a key difference. INTERACT tools are retrospective and provide a root-cause analysis of a readmission that has already occurred; the readmission becomes a case study to learn from so that the facility can prevent future readmissions. In contrast, the goal of predictive software is to identify a potential readmission before it becomes imminent.

Hospitals may view an SNF's reluctance to invest in predictive software as shortsighted and cheap and may think the SNF does not value the hospital as a partner in the coordinated care model. Hospitals will look to partner with SNFs that are willing to make the minimal investment in software that can extend the expertise of their nursing team and physicians to 24/7 monitoring of a patient's status.

Administrators who have invested in predictive software have told me it is a valuable tool. One administrator said he had not had one unnecessary readmission in more than six months since his team had implemented it. COMS Interactive (www.comsllc .com), the industry leader in this space, has started to partner with referring hospitals, health plans, assisted-living facilities, and home health providers to implement a common HIE. PointClickCare (www.pointclickcare.com) is another popular program.

For predictive software to succeed, the facility administrator and director of nursing of the facility implementing it must be firmly committed to it. Data from additional daily assessments may be required, and nurses may be reluctant to take on more tasks. Thus, the director of nursing must firmly believe in the importance and relevance of the predictive software and encourage the nursing staff to support the initiative.

In summary, SNFs must implement predictive software to better coordinate care. Although other tools are available to prevent readmissions, most are retrospective, not predictive. The SNF should educate its administrator, director of nursing, and other key nursing staff before implementing the software. Then the software should be rolled out with a comprehensive vision to share the data with staff and hospital referral sources to demonstrate the facility's commitment to preventing unnecessary readmissions. In addition, the SNF should deliver monthly readmission reports to its referring hospital partners and health plans as a way to distinguish its post-acute care facility as a preferred provider in the market.

ADOPT ADVANCING EXCELLENCE AND INTERACT TOOLS

In recent years, a number of tools have been specifically designed to help SNFs reduce readmissions. Two of the most common tools are Advancing Excellence and INTERACT. Although using both tools in an SNF may be repetitive and labor intensive, all SNFs should implement one or the other because the tools are vital in reducing an SNF's readmission rate and enabling the staff to identify key warning signs and indicators that often precede a hospital read-mission. If an SNF has not implemented these free tools, it risks being excluded from a hospital's list of preferred providers, narrow network, and transitional care program. Advancing Excellence and INTERACT are described in the two Perspectives that accompany this chapter.

IMPLEMENT DIRECT-FROM-ED AND OBSERVATION UNIT TRANSFERS

Although health plans have been using direct-from-ED and observation unit transfers as a tactic to reduce readmissions for many years, ED physicians have been hesitant to implement direct-to-SNF transfers without the direction of a health plan. Health plans provide three critical support mechanisms to make such transfers possible: aggressive case management, rapid discharge planning from the ED, and a comprehensive network of post-acute care facilities (to support the needs of these patients once discharged from the ED). Transfers directly from the ED to post-acute care were not mainstream in the fee-for-service era when hospitals and physicians were incentivized to admit patients because hospitals and health systems were often unable to commit to those three key concerns for ED physicians. However, in the post-ACA era, hospitals are penalized for admitting patients who could be cared for at a lower level of care, so transfers directly from the ED to post-acute care are becoming more common and will become the norm.

For many years, acute rehabilitation facilities have marketed to ED staff, educating them and advising them that acute rehabilitation facilities require only a physician order and not a prior acute hospital stay. In contrast, SNFs require a stay of three midnights (within the prior 30 days) before admission, and long-term acute care hospitals also have more conditions and benefit-specific requirements for transfer directly from the ED.

As the leading health systems pioneer new models to adapt to the ACA, it is becoming more common at all points of patient evaluation to aim to get the patient back home. If going home has been ruled out as an option, then other, lower levels of care should be considered before asking whether a patient needs to be admitted to an acute care hospital. Admission to an acute care hospital should be the last resort. Although more ED physicians will be using this approach, the transition is taking longer than many expected because most ED physician groups are still contracted and in some situations compensated by the hospital.

ED physicians and physician group leaders have traditionally been steered and guided by hospital administration. Because hospital administration has been slow to adapt to the many complexities of healthcare reform, ED physicians are largely stuck on the starting line as well. That said, transfers directly from the ED to post-acute care have arrived and will continue to grow as more and more healthcare organizations understand the financial implications and patient-centered model that is the ACA.

From a skilled-nursing provider's perspective, to best accommodate a request for a transfer from the ED, the facility needs to make sure that ED physicians, nurses, and case management staff have pertinent intake and admissions contact information for your SNF for both daytime and after hours. Furthermore, ED staff must know your facility's capabilities. INTERACT has an SNF capabilities tool that was designed for this purpose. Each facility is encouraged to complete the SNF capabilities form and deliver it regularly to hospital case managers and the ED so that they are aware of the clinical services the SNF provides.

Many hospitals collect data in their own spreadsheets and post a form in the ED showing the capabilities of each local skilled-nursing partner. Ideally, the spreadsheets also list the phone numbers of intake and the nursing station. This is important because in a post-ACA model, ED physicians and hospital administration are focused on shorter lengths of stay in the hospital and ED, so SNFs should be prepared to admit patients 24 hours a day.

After hours, SNFs may be tempted to turn away transfers if they cannot confirm whether Medicare days are available or need an authorization for coverage from the health plan. But in a post-ACA model, an SNF that wants to rise above the competition as the preferred provider will understand that most patients are eventually authorized for benefits or have available days. Therefore, admitting after hours without preconfirmation of Medicare benefits is a risk worth taking, particularly if the SNF strives to position itself as a preferred provider.

SNF marketers and admissions representatives should get to know ED physicians, nurses, and case managers because transfers directly from the ED to post-acute care will become a mainstream tactic to avoid unnecessary hospital stays. This opportunity for SNFs will require educating ED staff about your facility's skilled-nursing capabilities and willingness to admit after hours and on weekends.

Traditionally, hospitals considered observation status only for patients who might be candidates for transfer from the ED directly to an acute care facility. SNFs must educate ED physicians and staff that observation is not always the most appropriate placement for that patient—in a post-ACA model, an SNF can fill the role that observation previously played.

The next obvious question is, how will the SNF be compensated if the patient does not have three midnights in an acute care setting? This should not be a problem because any patient who is a readmission candidate in the ED has likely been in the hospital for three consecutive midnights in the past 30 days. As the model draws closer to an admission prevention mind-set, this three-midnight rule becomes more of a concern, but the three-midnight rule will likely be modified in some manner by the end of 2015.

CREATE A SECONDARY-MARKET SNF LIST

A skilled administrator will reach out to her secondary referring hospitals and encourage them to create a secondary-market SNF preferred provider list—a list of facilities that are not in the immediate surrounding area but are perhaps ten or more miles from the hospital. Although this tactic may produce only a handful of referrals from that hospital each year, sometimes that handful can make all the difference in terms of a facility's financial success.

Explain to the hospital that it is more at risk for readmissions when patients are referred to facilities outside their immediate area because they are not regularly communicating with them via a formal network or post-acute care network. Thus, a patient discharged from the hospital to a secondary-market SNF could be readmitted to another hospital multiple times and the original hospital that discharged the patient from the index stay might not ever know—yet this readmission would result in a penalty to the original hospital.

The solution is to encourage the hospital to create a secondary-market SNF preferred provider list or create a sample list for the hospital. Be sure to show why your facility is a preferred provider by mentioning the readmission prevention tactics you use, such as a POLST form for every patient and the INTERACT protocols. Also, showcase your monthly readmission data and commit to communicating with the hospital each time it sends you a patient. Finally, confirm that if a patient does need rehospitalization, you will return the patient to that hospital and not a different one. An effective nursing home administrator knows that hospitals want to retain market share as much as prevent readmissions and commits to making sure a patient returns to the original admitting hospital if acute care is needed. Hospitals still only get paid when a head is in a bed and are willing risk readmissions if they believe they will be reimbursed for a patient.

SUMMARY

Preventing readmissions in an SNF is critical for multiple reasons. Not only does it ensure the SNF remains in good standing with referring hospitals and physicians, but in 2017 SNFs will also begin to be penalized for unnecessary readmissions. The tactics in this chapter, if implemented effectively, can play a significant role in reducing an SNF's readmission rate and improving its reputation in the community.

PERSPECTIVE
Advancing Excellence in America's Nursing Homes: Tracking Tool and Resources for Safely Reducing Rehospitalizations

By Adrienne Mihelic, PhD
Senior biostatistician, Telligen Healthcare Intelligence

The Advancing Excellence in America's Nursing Homes Campaign was founded in 2006 by a coalition of 28 organizations, including nursing homes, government agencies, and quality improvement experts. Each state also has a Local Area Network for Excellence (LANE) to support the initiative.

The Advancing Excellence campaign supports those on the frontline of nursing home care with complete toolkits for nine quality goals, including the goal to safely reduce hospitalizations. The objective of this goal is to ensure that each and every transfer that occurs is medically justified and consistent with the resident's expressed preferences. Focusing on processes associated with transfers ensures that transfers occur as quickly as possible and with optimal continuity of care and communication.

To support the goal, the Advancing Excellence Safely Reduce Hospitalizations Tracking Tool and related resources were developed in conjunction with the INTERACT (Interventions to Reduce Acute Care Transfers) team and with support from the Centers for Medicare & Medicaid Services. The Advancing Excellence Safely Reduce Hospitalization Tracking Tool may be used to monitor implementation of INTERACT tools and transfer outcomes.

The Advancing Excellence Safely Reduce Hospitalizations package includes

- talking points;

$\rightarrow$

- fact sheets for residents and family, staff, and nursing home leadership;
- data tracking tools; and
- recommended interventions to improve the transition processes.

The materials are accessible to the public and free of charge. Many skilled-nursing facilities (SNFs) that are using the tools submit aggregate data monthly to establish baseline results for continued quality improvement. Although SNFs may display their own data, the initiative blinds all results, so specific SNFs are not identified. Those using the tool have access to written instructions, tutorials, and help desk support.

Other specific features of the Advancing Excellence tool include the following:

- Real-time data support data-driven quality improvement projects and documentation for additional nursing home quality projects.
- Graphs and charts provide actionable data, allowing a nursing home to evaluate patterns in transfer characteristics and monitor implementation of transfer-related processes.
- Charts and graphs may be customized for specific time periods.
- The data may be used in partnership with hospitals collaborating to reduce readmission rates.
- Charts and graphs are customizable to reflect the experience of residents admitted from a specific hospital.
- Monthly results are available for four transfer outcomes.
- The 30-day readmission rate and rates per 1,000 resident days are provided for transfers resulting in inpatient stay, transfers resulting in observation stay, and transfers resulting in an emergency department visit only.

$\longrightarrow$

◆ A matrix display of individual events can be scanned for patterns and daily flagging of residents who are still within the window for a 30-day readmission.

More information is available at www.nhqualitycampaign.org (on the website home page, select "Goals," and navigate to the Hospitalization goal area).

Note
This work, and the development of the Advancing Excellence Safely Reduce Hospitalizations Tracking Tool, was conducted by the Colorado Foundation for Medical Care, the Medicare Quality Improvement Organization for Colorado, under contract with the Centers for Medicare & Medicaid Services (CMS), an agency of the US Department of Health and Human Services (Contract Number HHSM-500-2008 CO9THC). The contents presented do not necessarily reflect CMS policy.

PERSPECTIVE
Interventions to Reduce Acute Care Transfers (INTERACT)

By David G. Wolf, PhD
CEO, INTERACT T.E.A.M. Strategies

Interventions to Reduce Acute Care Transfers (INTERACT), developed at Florida Atlantic University, is a publicly available quality improvement program designed to help skilled-nursing facilities (SNFs), assisted-living facilities, and home health care providers. The program offers best-practice tools, forms, guides, pathways, and tracking sheets designed to identify and manage acute changes in condition that would require a

→

patient's transfer to the emergency department. The result is a reduction in hospital readmissions in the SNF population.

INTERACT is recommended by the Centers for Medicare & Medicaid Services, and the tools are used by most SNFs in the United States. The program also helps long-term care facilities achieve compliance with the quality assurance performance improvement regulations established under Section 6102 of the Affordable Care Act as well as the Institute for Healthcare Improvement's Triple Aim of healthcare reform: improving care, improving health and satisfaction, and reducing costs.

The program is based on strategies in five fundamental areas:

1. Focus on principles of quality improvement. For example, implement the program with a team facilitated by a designated champion and given strong leadership support; measure, track, and benchmark clearly defined outcomes with feedback to all staff; and conduct root-cause analyses of hospitalizations to provide data for continuous learning and improvement.
2. Identify and evaluate changes in condition early—before they become severe enough to require hospital transfer.
3. When it is safe and feasible, manage common changes in condition without transferring the patient to the hospital.
4. Improve advance care planning and offer palliative or hospice care as an alternative to hospitalization when it is appropriate and when it is the choice of the resident or his healthcare proxy.

$\rightarrow$

5. Improve communication and documentation—within the SNF, between SNF staff and families, and between the SNF and the hospital.

More information about INTERACT may be found at the program's website (http://interact2.net).

CHAPTER 10

Preventing Readmissions in Long-Term Acute Care Hospitals and Acute Rehabilitation Hospitals

The Affordable Care Act (ACA) presents a conundrum for long-term acute care (LTAC) and acute rehabilitation hospitals. Although both types of specialty hospital are great alternatives for rehabilitating a patient who may not need acute hospitalization, a number of challenges prevent specialty hospitals from expecting significant growth in the post-ACA model.

As in other levels of post-acute care, quality outcomes, patient satisfaction, and profitable operations have always been the top three priorities for specialty hospitals. However, in a post-ACA era, preventing unnecessary hospital readmissions must be a key message point for those operating specialty hospitals, specifically LTAC and acute rehabilitation hospitals. A specialty hospital's ability to prevent unnecessary hospital readmissions will continue to be the means by which the facility sets itself apart from the others when being evaluated by its acute care referral partners. To be a preferred provider, LTAC and acute rehabilitation hospitals must succeed in several key areas:

- Quality care
- Patient satisfaction
- Accessibility (i.e., open beds should consistently be available)

- Ease of referral and discharge process
- Response to referral times
- Willingness to prioritize the payer's business initiatives and minimize those of the specialty (LTAC or acute rehabilitation hospital) model

And now, in the post-ACA era, one more key area should be added:

- Readmission prevention

Thus, the specialty hospital CEO's challenge in developing a readmission prevention strategy for his facility is making sure staff are trained to handle and care for as many clinical needs and situations as possible. The top priority of an operator in readmission prevention may be summed up as follows:

> The LTAC or acute rehabilitation hospital is responsible for preventing the patient from leaving the facility to return to a hospital.

Keep the patient in your facility whenever possible. Hospitals and health plans are not measuring specialty providers so much on their readmission rate as on their competency in caring for patients and not sending them to the emergency department (ED) unnecessarily. A specialty hospital CEO should take pride in the return-to-ED rate, not the return-to-acute-care rate.

Before reviewing readmission prevention tactics for specialty hospitals, some background is needed on how the ACA legislation affects specialty hospitals in general and LTAC and acute rehabilitation hospitals specifically.

SPECIALTY HOSPITALS

As a former hospital executive, I know that the acute care sector and those who operate acute care hospitals are not fans of specialty hospitals, including LTAC and acute rehabilitation hospitals. The reason is unclear, but it may be that because many providers of specialty services are large, publicly traded companies, they are perceived as prioritizing profitability over patient outcomes.

Including a chapter on specialty hospitals and their ability to provide solutions for readmission prevention would be irresponsible without discussing the financial aspect of the care provided at these facilities. On average, a typical per diem for an LTAC hospital ranges from $1,500 to $3,000. Although that may sound high for a post-acute care per diem, keep in mind that one of the reasons LTAC hospitals saw major growth in the 1990s and early 2000s was that this per diem often provided a significant savings over a normalized per diem for the same services in an acute-care hospital, which could range from $2,500 to $5,000.

Similarly, the per diem for an acute rehabilitation hospital has traditionally ranged from $900 to $1,800. Again, in comparison with with the normalized rates for acute care hospitals, significant savings can be achieved when a patient is discharged to an acute rehabilitation facility as an alternative to extending the length of stay in the acute care hospital.

However, per diem rates at specialty hospitals are notably higher than those at skilled-nursing facilities (SNFs), which range from $200 to $750. Considering that SNFs have increased their ability to care for patients with higher acuities in recent years, insurers and managed care organizations have turned almost exclusively to SNFs for post-acute care. In markets with more aggressive managed care organizations, it is unusual to find even one managed care preauthorization for LTAC or acute rehabilitation services in a year.

Although for years LTAC and acute rehabilitation hospital operators have marketed the higher level of care, increased quality results, and increased patient satisfaction offered by specialty hospitals, it all comes down to dollars and cents, and managed care organizations refuse to send patients to specialty hospitals if they think their needs can be met at an SNF. Specialty hospitals have also marketed to family members and physicians using an approach that appeals to the emotions of the patient and his family by saying they can avoid a nursing home or convalescent home for their loved one if they choose an LTAC or acute rehabilitation hospital.

Both LTAC and acute rehabilitation hospitals are licensed as hospitals, and they market this distinction aggressively because SNFs are not. Because LTAC and acute rehabilitation hospitals are licensed as specialty hospitals, they must meet all of the regulations for these types of hospitals to be licensed by the state in which they are located. In many cases, they provide services that SNFs cannot or that would require the SNF to obtain an additional license or certification.

The emergence of accountable care organizations and bundled-payment programs as a result of the ACA is a threat to specialty hospitals because insurers and health plans see specialty hospitals as higher-cost alternatives to care that could be provided at home or in an SNF. However, the biggest threat to specialty hospitals may be some of the other legislation that followed the passage of the ACA. Specifically, some states are absorbing all of the fee-for-service Medicare and Medicaid patients, referred to as "duals" (i.e., dually eligible for both benefits) into managed care organizations.

LTAC hospitals and acute rehabilitation providers experience a large decline in volume whenever post-acute care services require preauthorization from the insurer or health plan. Traditionally, specialty hospitals considered fee-for-service Medicare patients the bread and butter that drove their volume and profitability because these patients did not require preauthorization to be admitted. If the patient met the criteria for that type of specialty hospital, a physician's order was written and a transfer was facilitated.

Now that most dual patients will be managed by health plans and insurers, they will require preauthorization for post-acute care services by the insurer or health plan to ensure that they are being cared for responsibly and efficiently. Any patient who requires preauthorization for post-acute care services is more likely to be authorized for skilled nursing care or home health services than for care at a specialty hospital. This is almost entirely because of pricing and not necessarily because of quality results or service delivery.

For this reason, many companies have attempted to rebrand their LTAC hospitals as transitional care hospitals and are changing their overall business model to be more aggressive in the skilled nursing and home health service delivery areas. Other traditional LTAC hospital providers have forged partnerships with acute care providers and health plans to ensure that their business model remains viable in a post-ACA era. For example, Select Medical joined forces with UCLA Health System and Cedars-Sinai Medical Center to open a rehabilitation hospital in a vacant hospital building on the west side of Los Angeles (UCLA Health 2013).

The future appears increasingly challenging for specialty hospitals, including LTAC and acute rehabilitation hospitals, and payment reform is one issue under discussion. The conversations are being driven by the major specialty providers and the LTAC hospital and acute rehabilitation sector as a result of the challenges resulting from the ACA and other recent legislation. Momentum is swinging toward a single clinical tool that can be used at all levels of post-acute care and is tied to reimbursement levels.

Although LTAC hospitals and acute rehabilitation facilities have provided value-added services and filled a void in the post-acute care spectrum for many years, without major payment reform or the implementation of a single clinical tool tied to reimbursement for post-acute care providers, it will be difficult for LTAC hospitals and acute rehabilitation facilities to survive if all states force all their dual patients into managed care organizations. In short, post-acute care preauthorizations across the board would mean the death of the LTAC hospital and acute rehabilitation sectors as we know them.

LONG-TERM ACUTE CARE HOSPITALS

Specialty hospitals have proven to deliver quality outcomes and often are able to rehabilitate patients in a more cost-efficient manner than can be done in an acute care setting. Although LTAC hospitals have come under scrutiny in recent years because of the percentage of Medicare dollars being allocated for these bed days (as a fraction of overall Medicare bed days), LTAC hospitals in many markets continue to thrive despite significant legislative changes in recent years.

Several recent issues have made operating LTAC hospitals more difficult. LTAC hospitals are required to have an average length of stay of around 25 days for Medicare patients. This requirement has made them unpopular with their SNF counterparts because a long-term resident from an SNF might be hospitalized, transferred to an LTAC hospital, and then not return to the SNF for an additional 25 days. LTAC hospitals thrived in the 2000s and were not conscious of the negative reputation they were building among SNFs.

Then, when preauthorizations became the norm for post-acute care services for managed care and dual patients alike, health plans started making it more difficult to get authorization for LTAC hospital services. Between the 25-day requirement, lack of understanding of LTAC hospital services, and per diems that were three to four times bigger than those for an SNF, LTAC hospitals fell out of favor with health plans and managed care.

In a model that requires preauthorization of post-acute care services from the health plan or payer, LTAC hospitals and acute rehabilitation facilities are likely to suffer significant decreases in volume. In 2014, the federal government extended the moratorium on building new LTAC hospitals and tightened the rules for qualifying patients for LTAC hospital services, making the LTAC hospital business an even tougher proposition.

ACUTE REHABILITATION FACILITIES

Even before the passage of the ACA, the biggest advantage of acute rehabilitation hospitals over SNFs was their ability to admit patients directly from home. An acute rehabilitation admission requires only a physician's order, not a prior hospital stay, to be reimbursed by Medicare. Thus, one of the measurements acute rehabilitation operators use to assess growth and volume each month is the "admissions from home" category, which includes any patient admitted to the acute rehabilitation hospital who was not admitted directly from an acute care hospital.

Although this practice is not widespread, and admissions from home make up less than 15 percent of monthly readmissions in most acute rehabilitation facilities, the anticipated emergence of transfers directly from the ED to post-acute care suggests that acute rehabilitation facilities are well positioned to benefit from the practice. However, it will likely take a few years before transfers directly from the ED become the norm, and in the meantime, legislative changes will likely relax the three-midnight requirement for SNFs. If that is the case, acute rehabilitation facilities will have less of a chance to benefit from transfers directly from the ED.

No doubt more challenges than opportunities are ahead for acute rehabilitation hospitals as a result of the ACA. Acute rehabilitation hospitals will likely need to become even more specialized as they lose their traditional bread-and-butter patients—those being discharged from the hospital for rehabilitation services with the goal of returning home in two weeks. Most of those patients will be referred to skilled nursing or directly to home. As a result of this trend, acute rehabilitation facilities will be forced to elevate their level of services and become specialists in areas such as traumatic brain injury, spinal cord injury, cancer care, pediatric rehabilitation, post-stroke rehabilitation, amputee rehabilitation, and other specialty services. This level of specialization will require significant investment in specialized equipment and in continued education for nurses and therapists on how to best meet these patients' needs. Although acute rehabilitation facilities have provided quality care to patients, their business model is at risk because of recent legislation, and they will be forced to be creative if they are to continue to flourish in a post-ACA model.

The challenges facing acute rehabilitation and specialty hospitals in general should be kept in mind as they relate to the readmission prevention issue. Following are the readmission prevention tactics that build on those introduced in Part II, along with a brief description of how they should be applied in a specialty hospital setting.

MAKE SURE POLST FORMS ARE AVAILABLE FOR ALL PATIENTS

Specialty hospital leaders must make sure that every patient has a Physician Orders for Life-Sustaining Treatment (POLST) form in her chart at the nursing station. A copy of the POLST form should also be placed in a plastic sleeve and hung on or near the door in the patient's room so that if 911 emergency services are called or the patient is transported to the hospital, the paramedics can grab the plastic sleeve and take the POLST form with them to the hospital.

Nurses should always send a copy of the POLST form when the patient transfers to the hospital. For this reason, three copies of the POLST form should be inside the chart at all times because the hospital rarely sends it back when the patient returns to the specialty hospital.

CONDUCT OR GAIN ACCESS TO PATIENT RISK ASSESSMENTS

The specialty hospital is not necessarily responsible for performing patient risk stratifications, but caretakers at all levels must understand which patients are at high risk for readmission. The hospital and health system likely have significant resources and expensive tools to perform risk assessments, so the goal for specialty hospitals is to gain access to these risk tools to make sure caretakers are aware of high-risk patients when they arrive. Specialty hospitals should also have a protocol to raise staff awareness of high-risk patients.

PARTICIPATE IN POST-ACUTE CARE NETWORKS AND COMMUNITY COLLABORATIVES

All specialty hospital CEOs should seek out post-acute care networks and community collaboratives in their area. Many hospital-sponsored post-acute care networks may not include an LTAC hospital or acute rehabilitation facility. Be aware that this omission may be by design because the hospital knows its major insurers and health plan partners prefer not to refer to specialty hospitals. If this is the case in your market, consider it one more challenge to overcome. Continue to market to the hospital and ask case managers, physicians, and hospital leaders about different niches that your specialty hospital may be able to fill for difficult patients. Also, look for personnel changes in these positions as well as among hospitalists and in the C-suite, because new leaders may have a different perspective on specialty hospitals.

MAKE SURE YOU ARE PART OF THE HOSPITAL'S NARROW NETWORK

Hospitals are narrowing their networks. Instead of referring to all of the post-acute care providers in their region, they refer only to those they consider preferred providers.

Specialty hospitals must lobby to be in any narrow network. If your specialty hospital is not initially included in a narrow network, continue to reach out to the hospital and express your desire to be included. Often, your contacts at the hospital will be hesitant to say no to you because of an existing relationship. Most networks have a monthly, bimonthly, or quarterly meeting. At a minimum, ask to be invited to participate in the meetings even if the hospital does not consider you part of the network.

In summary, communicate and market to the hospital regularly, reach out to the C-suite to state your case, and engage physicians who are loyal to your facility and active at the hospital. In short, use any method you can to be included. Keep in mind that having a wide variety of health plan contracts will assist you in this process.

If it is a health plan or insurer that is narrowing the network, the issues identified here are still relevant. Regardless of who is narrowing the network, the specialty hospital operator needs to understand the goals of the narrow network and who is driving it, and work relentlessly to be included.

IDENTIFY LOCAL TRANSITIONAL CARE PROGRAMS

Specialty hospital operators should first identify which transitional care program is being used by the hospital or in the community, then read up on the specific program and make sure employees are prepared to fulfill their role in the process.

For example, several transitional care programs require a post-acute care follow-up visit to a primary care physician or high-risk patient clinic. Some hospitals ask the specialty hospital to schedule that appointment for after discharge from the specialty hospital. LTAC hospitals and acute rehabilitation facilities are under no obligation to do so, but complying with the request is a good way to stay in the hospital's good graces.

The specialty hospital may also consider pushing the hospital to connect with the specialty hospital electronically, creating a true community health information exchange (HIE). Because the acute care hospital or health system will likely not make this a priority, the LTAC hospital and acute rehabilitation facility should advocate for it.

PROVIDE AMBULATORY CASE MANAGEMENT SERVICES

Ambulatory case management refers to monitoring, servicing, and assisting the patient beyond discharge from the hospital, including beyond the specialty hospital stay. One of the benefits of narrowing the home health network is that it can manage this process on behalf of the specialty hospital.

However, when a patient discharged from the specialty hospital to home is not enrolled in a home health network, many hospitals look to the specialty hospital to provide a follow-up visit or place a phone call to the patient. Specialty hospitals that undertake home visits for their discharged patients are rare, so if a facility has the resources to provide this service consistently, this key differentiator would position the facility as a preferred provider with the referring hospital. At a minimum, however, the LTAC or acute rehabilitation hospital should place a follow-up call within 72 hours and another at the end of the first week after discharge.

PROVIDE REMOTE MONITORING SERVICES

Another way specialty hospitals can provide a higher level of care than that in SNFs is to partner with a hospital and physician to operate a remote monitoring unit. In many states, Medicare is now reimbursing for remote monitoring devices. When discharging a patient from the hospital, physicians can prescribe one of many different monitoring devices that will shorten hospital length of stay and allow the patient to return home sooner.

Many physicians have found that discharging patients to a specialty hospital that has specially trained nurses to monitor them is an even better solution. Providing remote monitoring services requires minimal investment from the specialty hospital. The monitoring is done at a central location staffed by operators who know whom to contact if the patient starts to decline. All specialty hospital providers should look into advances in remote monitoring technology and the companies that offer such services and educate physicians on how the technology may be used to shorten hospital length of stay and improve patient care.

COLLECT FACILITY-SPECIFIC DATA

A specialty hospital can never have enough data. Operators of LTAC and acute rehabilitation hospitals should know their facility's data. These data should be reviewed regularly by the facility's clinical staff and leadership team and with its hospital partners.

CONNECT VIA A HEALTH INFORMATION EXCHANGE

All specialty hospitals should be committed to connecting electronically with their key referral partners as soon as possible. Many hospitals and health systems have not yet reached out to post-acute care providers to connect via HIEs, but once the incentives and deadlines have passed for hospitals to implement electronic health records, hospitals will begin to look outward and realize the importance of connecting with their post-acute care providers.

LTAC hospitals and acute rehabilitation providers should not wait for the hospital to engage them in this conversation, however—they should start researching the hospital's connectivity requirements and software providers so that when the hospital is ready to have the discussion, they are prepared to quickly integrate.

HAVE A CONSISTENT MARKETING PLAN

LTAC hospitals and acute rehabilitation providers should develop a strategic and specific marketing plan as a means to connect with their referring hospital partners. Providing data about your facility should be a critical component of your marketing efforts. Monthly readmissions data are not typically available until around the tenth of the following month, so on the fifteenth of each month the specialty hospital's marketer should deliver an information package to each of his key contacts at the hospital.

The marketing package should include monthly readmission reports for that facility, remote monitoring success stories, and genetic test results for each patient referred from that hospital in the prior month. These data should be accompanied by a handwritten note from the marketer thanking the hospital for its business and noting his availability to answer any questions. The marketer should be sure to indicate that he will be back in touch on the fifteenth of the next month with new readmission data and genetic maps. A specialty hospital that consistently delivers these data each month will set itself apart from the others as a preferred provider that is committed to coordinated and patient-centered care.

PROMOTE SELF-MANAGEMENT, PATIENT HEALTH LITERACY, AND USE OF TEACH-BACK METHODS

Patient self-management is the most critical way to prevent readmissions at every level of care. Every specialty hospital operator should make sure that staff—particularly the director of nursing, nurses, nurse aides, social workers, therapists, and discharge planners—are all committed to educating patients to care for themselves.

The post-acute care provider's challenge is to understand the patient's home environment. No matter what the home environment is like, however, all patients need to learn to care for themselves, or else readmission is inevitable. To self-manage effectively, the patient must have a clear understanding of how to best care for her own needs.

Teach-back is the methodology most commonly used to ensure patient health literacy. In this patient-education method, the patient is provided with collateral material illustrating what he has learned and is then asked to confirm comprehension by reciting back or demonstrating the protocols he needs to self-administer his care. The specialty hospital should never underestimate its role in this process.

PURSUE CONTRACT ALIGNMENT

Given the focus on preventing readmissions and the national trend toward absorbing Medicare patients into managed care, it is more critical than ever that LTAC and acute rehabilitation hospitals have significant contract alignment. If a specialty hospital can find one or two health plans, insurers, or medical groups in its market that support it, those partners may be able to drive the specialty hospital's volume enough to offset the decline in volume that will result from other ACA initiatives.

Specialty hospitals should contract with any interested contract provider, even if it means accepting a lower reimbursement rate than is desirable. Times have changed, and the days of relying on Medicare reimbursement for financial viability are past.

CONDUCT GENETIC TESTING

Home health providers and SNFs have begun to see the value in ordering genetic tests to better manage their patients' medication regimens, reduce medication errors, and lower overall medication costs to the SNF. Genetic testing and DNA mapping are among the most important technological advances in recent years.

Genetic testing is now covered under Medicare Part B, and specialty hospital operators should study how implementing it can best meet the needs of the specialty hospital and its patients. This may mean working with physicians to order the genetic test on discharge if it is only covered as an outpatient benefit.

Many post-acute care providers have found that delivering copies of patients' genetic tests to the hospital each month differentiates the provider strategically from the competition. The referring hospital will recognize that the facility is leading the way and, after obtaining the proper consent, will appreciate being able to scan the report and summary into the patient's electronic health record for use by everyone connected to the HIE. Exhibit 9.1 (in Chapter 9) shows a sample genetic testing report.

NARROW THE HOME HEALTH NETWORK AND COORDINATE HOME HEALTH SERVICES

The specialty hospital must be a proactive partner in ensuring that a fluid transition exists for continued rehabilitation and therapy services if needed. Although a patient may not always need home health services after discharge from an LTAC hospital or acute rehabilitation facility, elderly patients should always be evaluated for home health services on discharge.

The ACA incentivizes providers to coordinate care to ensure a patient's well-being and avoid unnecessary hospital admissions. When a physician writes an order for home health services on discharge from any level of care, the order is for an evaluation. If the home health provider evaluates the patient in her home and determines that she is strong enough and well enough to care for herself in the absence of home health services, nothing is lost by having the evaluation done. Thus, all patients being discharged from a specialty hospital should be given a physician's order for a home health evaluation.

Specialty hospitals should also accept the fact that their acute care hospital partners have changed their home health referral patterns and are aggressively referring to a hospital-owned home health agency, partnering with a single home health agency, or narrowing their network of home health agencies. Specialty hospitals should know which home health agencies their key referring hospitals use and consider eliminating all other home health agencies it refers to other than those used by the hospital from which the patient was transferred.

ADOPT INTERACT TOOLS

INTERACT (Interventions to Reduce Acute Care Transfers) tools, which were designed for use in SNFs, can also be implemented in LTAC and acute rehabilitation hospitals (see http://interact2. net). Several INTERACT tools have been developed for specialty hospitals to improve their ability to coordinate care with acute care providers. If an LTAC or acute rehabilitation hospital has not implemented these free tools, it risks being excluded from a hospital's list of preferred providers, narrow network, and transitional care program.

IMPLEMENT DIRECT-FROM-ED AND OBSERVATION UNIT TRANSFERS

As leading health systems pioneer new models to adapt to the ACA, one increasingly common goal at all points of patient evaluation is to get the patient back home. If the patient is unable to return home, other lower levels of care should next be considered to avoid an acute care admission. This opens the door for a significant increase in transfers directly from the ED to post-acute care to avoid penalties for admitting patients who could be cared for at a lower level of care.

Although health plans have been using this tactic for many years, ED physicians are just starting to adopt this strategy for patients who are not managed by an insurer or health plan. This presents an opportunity for LTAC and acute rehabilitation hospitals.

To accommodate a request for a transfer from the ED, the specialty hospital needs to make sure ED physicians, nurses, and case management staff have pertinent intake and admissions contact information for the specialty hospital 24 hours a day. The ED staff must also know the specialty hospital's capabilities.

LTAC and acute rehabilitation hospital liaisons and marketers should get to know ED physicians, nurses, and case managers as transfers directly from the ED to post-acute care become a common tactic to avoid unnecessary hospital stays. To take advantage of this opportunity, specialty hospitals need to educate ED staff on the facility's capabilities and market the facility's willingness to admit from the ED after hours and on weekends.

SUMMARY

The tactics discussed in this chapter and in the accompanying Perspective shed light on the importance of remaining in good standing with your hospital referral sources by implementing tools to prevent unnecessary readmissions. The ACA has made operating an LTAC or acute rehabilitation hospital even tougher from a reimbursement standpoint, so it is more important than ever that operators of these facilities implement effective readmission prevention protocols.

PERSPECTIVE
Using Post-Acute Care Venues to Reduce Readmissions

By Cherilyn G. Murer, JD
President and CEO, Murer Consultants Inc.

According to the Centers for Medicare & Medicaid Services, approximately 40 percent of Medicare hospital discharges are to another venue of care (Gage et al. 2012). Three of the primary venues following discharge are skilled-nursing facilities (SNFs), inpatient rehabilitation facilities (IRFs), and long-term acute care (LTAC) hospitals. With the onset of readmission penalties, hospitals must focus greater attention on the venues used after patient discharge to prevent avoidable readmissions.

Effective care transition and an improved care continuum are two key factors in readmission prevention. Through close partnerships with SNFs, IRFs, and LTAC hospitals, general hospitals in the inpatient prospective payment system can ensure that their patients receive quality care at a venue providing acuity-intensive services at a lower level. Post-acute care venues provide many benefits to reduce readmissions, but some challenges must be addressed.

Benefits
The immediate benefit a post-acute care venue offers is that the patient will spend fewer days in the hospital. Fewer days in the hospital diminishes the likelihood of a hospital-acquired infection and significantly reduces the likelihood of readmission (Emerson et al. 2012). Although a patient spends fewer days in the hospital, once he is in an SNF, IRF, or LTAC hospital, he will continue to receive substantial nursing care that will be more attentive to his needs because these venues are able to provide nursing care that can be more easily tailored to helping transition the patient home. →

Post-acute care venues provide a more stable continuum of care for patients and help prevent patients from being lost in the shuffle. A significant number of readmissions are the result of patients failing to adhere to postdischarge instructions (Watson et al. 2011), and post-acute care venues help prevent that. In addition, many readmissions result from patients not knowing where to go or having limited care options available in the event of a perceived health crisis. Post-acute care institutions are capable of managing those events within the post-acute care setting rather than the patient presenting at an emergency department and likely being readmitted to a hospital. Many post-acute care venues have procedure rooms where they can provide many of the same services as the emergency department of a general acute care hospital.

Challenges

Post-acute care venues face two primary challenges related to readmission. The first is effective communication of the patient's care/discharge plan between the hospital and the post-acute care venue. The second is making physicians comfortable with using the full clinical capabilities that post-acute care venues offer.

Often, readmissions from a post-acute care venue result when the hospital's discharge plan does not reach or is not fully understood by the post-acute care venue (King et al. 2013). In many cases, something regarding the patient's treatment plan is lost in translation, leading to the patient's suffering an acute event and being readmitted. The lapse in communication cannot necessarily be attributed to either provider because the hospital and the post-acute care venue should work as a team to ensure effective communication.

→

Beyond the challenge of effective communication, physicians often drive readmissions from a post-acute care venue. Physicians have cited two main reasons for a hospital admission from an SNF: (1) The physicians thought the on-site capabilities of the SNF were not sufficient to address patients' medical issues, and (2) the physicians were "more comfortable" with the services provided in the hospital setting, specifically rapid laboratory results, imaging capabilities, and nursing staff competencies (Perry et al. 2010). These factors indicate that many physicians struggle with using and relying on the capabilities of post-acute care venues.

Solutions
First and foremost, hospitals and post-acute care venues can improve patient care and prevent unnecessary readmissions by recognizing that they are partners in this challenge and working together to strengthen the lines of communication. Partnered providers should collectively agree on standard care transition plans and standard policies to ensure that patients and their treatment plans do not fall through the cracks. Ideally, post-acute care venues would work with the hospital in the discharge planning process and also perform their own preadmission assessment to identify any potential risk factors that would increase the likelihood of readmission. Patients identified as high risk should receive increased attention from the nursing staff.

After admission, post-acute care venues should perform medication reconciliation with the primary care physician to confirm that there are no conflicting medications (or other errors) between the hospital's discharge plan and the medication the patient was on before hospital admission. Post-acute care venues should be proactive and use tools

$\rightarrow$

to track their own readmission data, ideally both daily and monthly. The daily tool should be used as a means of root-cause analysis to promote rapid problem resolution, and the monthly tool should be used to track overall readmission trends that will permit the provider to recognize potential skill deficits within the nursing units. Other key factors in preventing readmissions are physician coverage and support; nursing staff levels, competencies, and turnover rates; and facility capabilities, including the availability of laboratory, pharmacy, and imaging services.

Conclusion
Reducing unnecessary readmissions is a challenge that all providers across the continuum of care must work together to address. Through proper utilization of post-acute care venues and effective management of those venues, the quality of care patients receive will improve and readmissions will decline.

REFERENCES

Emerson, C. B., L. M. Eyzaguirre, J. S. Albrecht, A. C. Comer, A. D. Harris, and J. P. Furuno. 2012. "Healthcare-Associated Infection and Hospital Readmission." *Infection Control and Hospital Epidemiology* 33 (6): 539–44.

Gage, B., M. Morley, L. Smith, M. J. Ingber, A. Deutsch, T. Kline, J. Dever, J. Abbate, R. Miller, B. Lyda-McDonald, C. Kelleher, D. Garfinkel, J. Manning, C. M. Murtaugh, M. Stineman, and T. Mallinson. 2012. *Post-Acute Care Payment Reform Demonstration: Final Report.* RTI Project Number 0209853.005.001. Published March. www.cms.gov /Research-Statistics-Data-and-Systems/Statistics-Trends-and

-Reports/Reports/Research-Reports-Items/PAC_Payment
_Reform_Demo_Final.html.

King, B. J., A. L. Gilmore-Bykovskyi, R. A. Roiland,
B. E. Polnaszek, B. J. Bowers, and A. J. H. Kind. 2013.
"The Consequences of Poor Communication During
Hospital to Skilled Nursing Facility Transitions: A Qualitative
Study." *Journal of the American Geriatrics Society* 61 (7):
1095–102.

Perry, M., J. Cummings, G. Jacobson, T. Neuman, and J.
Cubanski. 2010. *To Hospitalize or Not to Hospitalize? Medical
Care for Long-Term Care Facility Residents.* Henry J. Kaiser
Family Foundation. Published October. https://kaiser
familyfoundation.files.wordpress.com/2013/01/8110.pdf.

UCLA Health. 2013. "Cedars-Sinai, UCLA Health System and
Select Medical Plan to Open Rehabilitation Hospital."
Published December 3. www.uclahealth.org/body.cfm?id=561
&action=detail&ref=2341.

Watson, A. J., J. O'Rourke, K. Jethwani, A. Cami, T. A. Stern,
J. C. Kvedar, H. C. Chueh, and A. H. Zai. 2011. "Linking
Electronic Health Record–Extracted Psychosocial Data in
Real-Time to Risk of Readmission for Heart Failure."
Psychosomatics 52 (4): 319–27.

CHAPTER 11

Preventing Readmissions
in Home Health Agencies

After the Affordable Care Act (ACA) was passed in 2010, home health providers celebrated the opportunity ahead. They believed the ACA would make home health an even more lucrative business than it had been under the fee-for-service model. With the ACA's six different programs that incentivized health systems and hospitals to reduce readmissions, coordinate care, and admit only patients who could not be cared for at a lower level of care, it appeared initially as if home health services would to continue to grow in the post-ACA era.

Although the ratio and volume of home health referrals and patients will likely increase over what was the norm during the fee-for-service era, the aggressive thinning in the number of home health agencies was completely unexpected. So in essence, volume will grow but some providers will disappear. Many hospitals have created transitional care programs that are a means of funneling as many patients as possible into their own home health agency in the effort to better coordinate care and align with the ACA. Hospitals and health systems that do not own their own home health agency have begun narrowing their network to five or fewer home health agencies in an effort to better coordinate care.

Although many hospitals had their own home health agency in the 1990s, the early 2000s brought a wave of closures because it was difficult to post a profit in the home health service line and there did not appear to be any reward for the hospitals to continue operating home health agencies. Furthermore, a hospital system's overhead was often too high to operate a profitable home health agency; freestanding agencies had much lower costs and overhead than hospital-based agencies did. In the next few years, however, hospitals and health systems will likely get back into the home health business. Those that do not wish to get back into the business as operators may consider a joint venture or narrow their network to one provider. Hospitals have an opportunity to create a new revenue stream because the ACA has opened the door for them to drive significant volume to their own home health agency through such creative means as a transitional care program.

The issue of choice and antisteering regulations is relevant here. Those laws were put into place to prevent inappropriate financial arrangements between physicians, facility operators, and their post-acute care partners. The ACA is an almost complete reversal of those regulations. If hospitals and health systems do not coordinate care with post-acute care providers, they will be penalized and their reimbursement will be withheld or recovered. Therefore, the table is set for hospitals and health systems to operate their own post-acute care services—with the biggest opportunity being in home health.

Ambulatory case management has a role in home health services. In essence, ambulatory case management comes down to one of two tactics: home visits or telephone calls. Home visits are an expense to the health system unless a patient is receiving home health services. To carry this idea further, Medicare and private insurers reimburse the provider (health system or agency) for home health services. Thus, if home health nurses, therapists, and other staff are trained to identify risk factors and ask basic follow-up questions, the health system has a means to be reimbursed for monitoring its patients while continuing their therapy and rehabilitative process through home health services. To use a cliché, they can kill two birds with one stone. Consider how valuable this service would be in the case of high-risk patients. The health system would be responsible for paying a nurse or caretaker to go into the patient's home to monitor him in any situation other than if the patient were already receiving home health services.

Thus, a health system–owned home health agency should make sure its caretakers are trained to assess and document the same issues and risk factors that an ambulatory case manager would. Home health agencies that are not owned by the health system, whether part of the narrow network or not, should also be training their entire team to serve in this capacity.

Given the overlap, should home health agency owners talk to health systems and hospitals about partnering to do their ambulatory case management while they are providing home health services? I am not aware of this happening in many instances beyond specific transitional care programs designed for this reason. However, many innovative home health agency owners have designed specialty programs. CareCentrix, for example, is a leader in providing value-added services in the home health sector. For many years it has contracted with several major health plans to bring a higher level of care to their home health patients. CareCentrix has an innovative model: They are not a provider of home health services but a management company that provides support services to enhance coordinated care tools for home health providers.

Although quality will always be the first requirement of any post-acute care provider a hospital will refer to, a home health agency must get a few other factors right to be considered a provider of choice or preferred provider. To be a preferred home health provider, an agency must succeed in several key areas:

+ Quality
+ Patient satisfaction

- Ease of referral and discharge process
- Response to referral times

And now, in the post-ACA era, two more key areas should be added:

- Readmission prevention
- Ambulatory case management (be the eyes and ears in the home, looking for risk factors)

With this in mind, the administrator's challenge in developing a readmission prevention strategy for her home health agency is making sure staff are trained to observe for risk factors, communicate with the patient, prepare patients to self-manage, ensure patient health literacy, practice teach-back methods, and fulfill all other roles of the ambulatory case manager. A home health agency's top priority in preventing readmissions may be summed up as follows:

> The home health agency is responsible for ensuring that a patient continues to rehabilitate at home and does not return to the hospital unnecessarily. Further, a home health care team member must act as an ambulatory case manager by ensuring that the home is safe and free of risk factors.

In short, keep the patient at home whenever possible. Health systems and insurers are not measuring home health agencies so much on their readmission rate as on their competency in caring for patients and not sending them to the emergency department (ED) unnecessarily. Thus, a health agency provider should focus on the return-to-ED rate, not the return-to-acute-care rate.

Once a patient is in the ED, the home health agency has no control over readmission because the hospital makes the readmission decision. Thus, the home health agency administrator should manage the situation at his end by being aware of every patient who leaves for any reason to go to any hospital. When the agency administrator makes this a priority, discusses all return-to-ED patients every morning with the home health team, and shows a consistent commitment to preventing unnecessary readmissions, an agency culture of preventing unnecessary ED visits will follow.

In the fee-for-service model, when a patient receiving home health services started to decline, a nurse would tell the physician, and the physician's response was to send the patient to the ED. This response was not only convenient for the physician but also the safest approach. In addition, in a fee-for-service model the physician, the hospital, and the home health agency (because it likely justified an extended service episode) gained a financial benefit each time a patient was readmitted to the hospital.

Following are readmission prevention tactics that build on those introduced in Part II, along with a brief description of how they should be applied in a home health agency setting.

MAKE SURE POLST FORMS ARE AVAILABLE FOR ALL PATIENTS

Home health agencies must make sure that every patient has a Physician Orders for Life-Sustaining Treatment (POLST) form in her chart. A copy of the POLST form should also be placed in a plastic sleeve and hung on or near the door of the patient's home so that if 911 emergency services are called or the patient is transported to the hospital, the paramedics can grab the plastic sleeve and take the POLST form with them to the hospital.

Nurses should always send a copy of the POLST form when the patient transfers to the hospital. For this reason, three copies of the POLST form should be inside the chart at all times because the hospital rarely sends it back when the patient returns home.

CONDUCT OR GAIN ACCESS TO PATIENT RISK ASSESSMENTS

The home health agency is not necessarily responsible for performing patient risk stratifications, but it is critical for caretakers at all levels to understand which patients are at high risk for readmission. The hospital and health system likely have significant resources and expensive tools to perform risk assessments, so the home health agency's goal should be to gain access to these risk tools so that caretakers are aware of high-risk patients when they begin home health services. Additionally, home health agencies should have a protocol for high-risk patients, at a minimum to raise awareness that the patient is a "frequent flyer" to the hospital. A variety of protocols may be used to identify high-risk patients, but the important point is that the agency must have a protocol, and the agency's leadership must communicate its importance.

PARTICIPATE IN POST-ACUTE CARE NETWORKS AND COMMUNITY COLLABORATIVES

Every home health agency should seek out post-acute care networks or community collaboratives in their area. The topics of the meetings are not nearly as important as your presence there. If your agency does not show up to the meeting, it sends a message to the hospital that readmissions are not a priority and the hospital is not an important referral source.

If the hospitals that refer to you do not have their own post-acute care network and there is no community collaborative, consider taking the lead in forming a community collaborative. If a hospital limits its post-acute care network to skilled-nursing facilities (SNFs), make sure you know which facilities those are so that you can target your marketing efforts to them.

MAKE SURE YOU ARE PART OF THE HOSPITAL'S NARROW NETWORK

Home health agencies must position themselves and lobby to be in any narrow network. Hospitals are narrowing their networks, and rather than referring to all of the home health agencies in their region, they refer to only a few preferred providers (Exhibit 11.1).

Although this practice seems antithetical to patient choice and anti-steering regulations, the ACA incentivizes hospitals to narrow their network and penalizes them if they do not. Patient choice and anti-steering regulations remain in place, but hospitals have found creative ways to steer patients to their post-acute care facilities and providers of choice while still allowing patients to believe they had a choice.

Exhibit 11.1 How Hospitals Are Narrowing Their Home Health Providers

Centers for Medicare & Medicaid Services (CMS)–Required Comprehensive List of Home Health Agencies

Hospital's CMS-required list of all home health agencies in the area

Hospital's Post-Acute Care Network List of Home Health Agencies

One to five agencies selected by the hospital
for its post-acute care network

Hospital's Transitional Care Program List of Home Health Agencies

---

Home health administrators should not waste time worrying about whether it is legal or appropriate if a hospital takes such action. Instead, spend your energy making sure your agency is one of the preferred providers in the narrow network.

If the hospital owns a home health agency, then the hospital will likely include only its own hospital-based agency in the narrow network. If the hospital does not own a home health agency, then it will likely include no more than three home health agencies in the transitional care program so that it can manage them more closely.

IDENTIFY LOCAL TRANSITIONAL CARE PROGRAMS

Home health agency operators should first identify which transitional care program is being used by the hospital or in the community, then read up on the specific program and make sure employees are prepared to fulfill their role in the process.

For example, several transitional care programs require a post-acute care follow-up visit to a primary care physician or high-risk patient clinic. Some health systems have started asking the home health agency to serve as an ambulatory case manager, as their eyes and ears in the home, and to schedule the follow-up appointment after discharge from the hospital or SNF. Although home health agencies are under no obligation to do so, complying with the request is one way to stay in the hospital's good graces.

PROVIDE AMBULATORY CASE MANAGEMENT SERVICES

Ambulatory case management refers to the task of monitoring, servicing, and assisting the patient beyond discharge from the hospital to an SNF. One of the benefits of narrowing the home health network is that it can manage the process on behalf of the hospital and SNF.

The main goals of an ambulatory case management home visit are to

- confirm that the patient has safely transferred to his living environment,
- ensure that the patient understands his medication regimen and has an adequate supply of medication,
- ensure that the patient is comfortable and not anxious about self-management or his living environment, and
- identify risk factors visually on a home visit or through questions on a phone call.

Clearly, it makes sense for the home health service provider to fulfill this role, and it may be the most important value-added service health systems and payers consider when choosing a home health provider. That is, agencies that are willing to spend a few extra minutes each day doing ambulatory case management on behalf of the patient will be given consideration by the payer.

As another way to stand above the competition, many home health agencies are notifying hospitals and primary care physicians as a courtesy when a patient is discharged from the SNF to home, specifically patients within the 30-day discharge window (often, the physician is unaware that a hospitalist and SNF handled the patient). An agency might consider taking it a step further by including in the hospital notification a plan to update the hospital on the patient's 72-hour postdischarge visit and then again a week later. Doing so will position your agency as a preferred provider over the competition.

PROVIDE REMOTE MONITORING SERVICES

A great way for home health agencies to set themselves apart from their competition is to partner with a hospital and physician to support remote monitoring services. In many states, Medicare is now reimbursing for remote monitoring devices. When discharging a patient from the hospital, a physician can prescribe one of many different monitoring devices that will shorten the hospital length of stay and allow a patient to return home from the hospital sooner.

The investment required of the home health agency to provide remote monitoring services is minimal and is mainly related to education of care team members. The devices use wireless technology, and monitoring is usually done at a central location staffed by operators who know whom to contact if the patient starts to decline.

COLLECT FACILITY-SPECIFIC DATA

Knowledge is power. Know your home health agency data, and know it as soon as possible because Centers for Medicare & Medicaid Services reports are often delayed by more than a year. Whether you partner with a software provider or collect the data on your own, having these data each month is imperative.

The data should be reviewed by your clinical staff and leadership team and should also be shared with your hospital partners. If you are hesitant to share data with your hospital partners, perhaps you have some work to do on the quality side.

CONNECT VIA A HEALTH INFORMATION EXCHANGE

All home health agencies should be committed to connecting electronically with their key referral partners as soon as possible. Many hospitals and health systems have not yet reached out to post-acute care providers to connect via health information exchanges (HIEs), but once the incentives and deadlines have passed for hospitals to implement electronic health records, hospitals will begin to look outward and realize the importance of connecting with their post-acute care providers.

An HIE will be particularly important if the hospital migrates toward a discharge-to-home mind-set and narrows its network of home health agencies to help it bring this vision to fruition. Home health agency operators should not wait for the hospital to engage them in this conversation, however—they should start researching hospital's connectivity requirements and software providers, so that when the hospital is ready to have the discussion, the agency is prepared to quickly integrate.

HAVE A CONSISTENT MARKETING PLAN

Home health agencies can benefit from more consistent marketing to referral sources and should develop a strategic and specific marketing plan that includes monthly data distribution to these referral sources. Monthly data are typically not available until around the tenth of the following month, so on the fifteenth of each month the home health marketer should deliver an information package to each of her key contacts at the hospital and SNF. The information package should include monthly readmission reports, remote monitoring success stories, and genetic test results and case summaries for each patient referred from that source in the prior month. The package should be accompanied by a handwritten note from the marketer thanking the contact for his business and noting the marketer's availability to answer any questions. The marketer should be sure to indicate that she will be back in touch on the fifteenth of the next month with new readmission data and genetic maps. Consistency speaks volumes to referral sources.

Another marketing strategy is to notify the hospital when a patient is successfully transitioned home without a readmission within 30 days of the index stay. This simple action shows great consideration for your referral source. Consider celebrating the achievement by sending the hospital a congratulatory e-mail, letter, or certificate on behalf of the care coordination team with language such as the following:

> On behalf of the Hometown Home Health Agency, we would like to thank you for trusting us with the care of patient F. Smith. We are writing to advise you that Mr. Smith transitioned home safely under the care of our home health agency. It has been 30 days since he was discharged from your hospital, and we are pleased to inform you that he has not been readmitted to any hospital. Thank you again for trusting us with the care of this patient. We appreciate your partnership and shared commitment to quality and preventing avoidable readmissions.

The home health marketer could also send this certificate or letter (on agency letterhead, of course) to the physician's office and to the hospital case management team. Although I do not know of any home health agencies using this tactic, delivering such letters would be a powerful way for an agency to distinguish itself from others.

PROMOTE SELF-MANAGEMENT, PATIENT HEALTH LITERACY, AND USE OF TEACH-BACK METHODS

Patient self-management is the most critical way to prevent readmissions at every level of care. Every home health agency should make sure that all staff are committed to educating patients to care for themselves.

The ultimate goal is to get the patient home safely, and the post-acute care provider's challenge is to understand the patient's home environment. No matter what the home environment is like, however, all patients need to learn to care for themselves or else readmission is inevitable. Patient health literacy is necessary for effective self-management. In short, the patient must have a clear understanding of how to best care for her own needs.

Teach-back is the patient-education method most commonly used to ensure patient health literacy. The patient is provided with collateral material illustrating what she has learned and is then asked to confirm her comprehension by reciting back or demonstrating the protocols she needs to self-administer her care. The home health agency caretaker should never underestimate his role in this process.

If the home health agency hopes to be included in a narrow network and be viewed as a preferred provider, it must take an active, calculated role in fulfilling the educational mission of the transitional care program, post-acute care network, or community collaborative. Ignoring this piece of the process and assuming that the acute care hospital, health plan, and SNF will ensure patient health literacy would be naive and short-sighted for a home health agency.

PURSUE CONTRACT ALIGNMENT

Given the focus on preventing readmissions and the national trend toward absorbing Medicare patients into managed care, it is more critical than ever that home health agencies have significant contract alignment. As the ACA has largely shifted the influence away from the hospital and physician in the coordinated care model, health plans and insurers have gained even more influence in the process. Thus, all home health agencies should aggressively seek contracts and no longer rely on Medicare patients to cover the cost of operations.

CONDUCT GENETIC TESTING

One of the most important technological advances in recent years is the availability of DNA testing and genetic mapping. Home health agencies have begun to see the value in ordering genetic tests to better manage patients' medication regimens, reduce medication errors, and lower overall medication costs.

The procedure, which is covered by Medicare Part B as of January 1, 2014, may be conducted once in a patient's lifetime. The hospital community has been slow to order genetic maps because the benefit is not approved under Medicare Part A and hospitals are not reimbursed for inpatients. Many home health agencies, however, recognize that genetic testing not only is a means to improve patient care but also gives them a marketing advantage over their competitors. Thus, they have begun ordering these tests for their patients and (after obtaining the proper consent) sharing the results with the referring hospital partner to be scanned into the electronic health record for permanent use.

The most important thing for home health agencies to remember about genetic testing is that it is in the best interest of the patient and will reduce the overall costs of providing care—outcomes that are consistent with the goals of the ACA. In addition, a commitment to genetic testing will distinguish an agency from its competition and mark it as an innovative partner in the coordinated care model. As noted earlier in this chapter, delivering genetic test results to the hospital is an effective marketing strategy. The hospital will appreciate being able to scan the report and summary into the patient's electronic health record for use by everyone connected to the health information exchange. (See Exhibit 9.1 in Chapter 9 for a sample genetic testing report.)

ADOPT INTERACT TOOLS

INTERACT (Interventions to Reduce Acute Care Transfers) offers several free tools that home health agencies can use to improve their ability to coordinate care with acute care providers (see http://interact2.net). If a home health agency has not implemented these tools, it risks being excluded from a hospital's list of preferred providers, narrow network, and transitional care program.

TRIAGE THE PATIENT WHEN AN ACUTE CARE EPISODE OCCURS

When an acute episode occurs, it is critical that the home health agency take immediate action to avoid a readmission. Thus, when a patient under your service calls, do not automatically send her to the ED. If it is not an emergency, the patient can be referred to another resource that meets her specific need. Actions the agency can take include the following:

- Refer the patient to her primary care physician's office.
- Send the patient to an urgent care clinic.
- Have the patient visit the post-acute care clinic.
- Send a home health nurse or therapist to the patient's home.
- Have the patient or caregiver contact a pharmacist to answer medication questions.
- Contact a family member to provide support or a second opinion.
- Transfer the patient directly to the SNF, long-term acute care hospital, or acute rehabilitation hospital if the patient was discharged from the hospital in the prior 30 days.

If the situation is not an emergency, the goal is to contact someone who can provide the necessary information, help, or comfort to the patient while avoiding an unnecessary hospital readmission.

REFER ALL PATIENTS TO HOME CARE OR PRIVATE-DUTY NURSING ON DISCHARGE

Once a patient is discharged from home health services, she has reached the symbolic finish line of that episode of care. Thus, the discharge from home health services to a home caretaker or private-duty nurse represents the handoff between post-acute care and a healthy lifestyle (or wellness). Discharging a patient from home health services indicates that he has reached full recovery or has plateaued and can no longer benefit from home health services or is no longer covered for home health services.

At this point in the recovery process, Medicare or the insurer ceases to reimburse providers. Although a patient may continue to receive therapy on an outpatient basis or visit a physician's office for a specific need, once the home health episode concludes, any home-based care has to be paid for by the patient because the insurer is no longer responsible. Despite the lack of reimbursement, it is a good practice to encourage at-risk patients who are being discharged from home health services to arrange for continued support from a home care provider or private-duty nurse. Because the patient pays for such services, a physician's order is not required. Of course, the patient can and often does refuse services, but the health system, health plan, or payer has nothing to lose by encouraging every patient to consider such support services.

The home care provider or private-duty nurse can serve as a de facto ambulatory case manager in the postdischarge period to ensure the patient's continued well-being and minimize risk factors. Though no longer financially responsible, the health system, health plan, or insurer continues to benefit from the caretakers serving as eyes and ears in the home.

IMPLEMENT TRANSFERS DIRECTLY FROM THE ED TO HOME WITH HOME HEALTH SERVICES

Many healthcare leaders assume that patients are discharged from the ED to home with an order for home health services. However, this was rare in the fee-for-service model, where physicians and hospitals were incentivized to admit patients. In the post-ACA model, direct transfers from ED to home will become a common practice requiring only a minor tweak in a hospital's ED case management delivery. In short, hospitals and health systems must make sure their ED case managers are equipped to discharge patients home with a home health evaluation order to eliminate liability concerns.

SUMMARY

The days when a home health agency could hire a physician as medical director to bolster referrals and volume are rapidly coming to an end. If your agency is not part of a narrow network, then its future is already in jeopardy. More so than in any other sector, the home health delivery model will completely change as a result of the ACA. This chapter and its accompanying Perspective provide a number of tactics that can be implemented to reduce readmissions and ensure that your agency is well positioned to be included in a narrow network.

The home health model of the past was lucrative, but the home health model of the future is the narrow network, meaning a few high-quality agencies with higher volumes and lower margins. Agencies that align with the payer, deliver quality results, and accept a lower margin in return for higher volume (contracts often include volume guarantees) will continue to thrive. Agencies that remain stuck in the fee-for-service free-for-all mentality and attempt to use the marketing tactics of the past to generate volume and revenue will likely wither and die. Home health agency operators can no longer use old-school tactics to work around the hospital or health system's current efforts to narrow their network. Agencies that refuse to adapt to a coordinated care approach (and thereby promote the outward migration of the referring hospital's coordinated care model) will be vulnerable—and will likely go out of business.

Adapt, conform, and join the narrow network. Serve as an ambulatory case manager, be the eyes and ears of the care team looking for risk factors in the home, and confirm that the patient understands the care plan and medication regimen. Ensure that the patient has an ample supply of medication, and celebrate when the patient has successfully transitioned home without a readmission within 30 days of the index stay. All of these tactics will set your home health agency apart from the others in a post-ACA model.

PERSPECTIVE
Rehabilitation Is Vital in Readmission Prevention

By Sarah Thomas
Rehabilitation specialist and legislative affairs liaison,
Hallmark Rehabilitation, San Francisco

With increasing financial pressures and national attention, hospitals are being compelled to focus on reducing readmission rates. This focus has generated an increase in solution-driven initiatives. The greater challenge, however, is to shift this focus to serve as a catalyst to create patient-driven initiatives. Attention to the patient-centered model of care is imperative to the readmission prevention process. Many key players in this paradigm shift are working to improve fluid communication and seamless transitions. The patient-centered service delivery model should transcend individual practice areas and settings. Continuity of care and comprehensive collaboration are essential.

Often overlooked and underrepresented in the discussion of readmission prevention is the vital role of rehabilitation across the care continuum. Physical and occupational therapists and speech language pathologists address the daily challenges patients face during all phases of care. Multidisciplinary rehabilitation teams assess and provide therapeutic intervention at hospitals, acute rehabilitation centers, and along the post-acute care continuum at skilled-nursing facilities (SNFs), assisted-living facilities, and home care and outpatient levels. Rehabilitation must be a constant thread woven into the fabric of the care continuum.

→

Rehabilitation professionals bring a patient-centered approach to intervention that addresses the physical, cognitive, social-emotional, and environmental factors patients are challenged with when facing illness or injury. Many factors affecting a person's well-being are addressed by rehabilitation therapy professionals. For example, a procedure performed at the hospital must be fully understood by the rehabilitation team at every level of care. They must assess how the procedure and any underlying comorbidities may affect the patient's ability to safely return home and perform her daily tasks. They assess what level of care or intervention will be needed for the patient to function safely in a transitional environment and what is needed to improve to his prior level of function. The rehabilitation team evaluating at the hospital has a role to clearly communicate to the receiving team what the immediate and ongoing care needs are for the patient at the next level of care. Communication is crucial across the continuum.

If the patient is to return home, the therapists at the hospital must first assess a myriad of things: the patient's overall functional status, ability to communicate, and ability to comprehend and execute cognitively demanding tasks; the ability of family members to safely support the community reentry; the need for adaptive equipment or devices to improve safety and function; and so on. The care team at home, including the therapists, will need to thoroughly review all documentation to be certain the continuity of care is seamless. Case management, nursing, and social services are often prioritized upon discharge home. Therapists also play a vital role in this transition. The rehabilitation team's assessment and modification of the home environment, therapeutic intervention, and patient/caregiver education are all important components of a successful transition home. The rehabilitation team helps to prevent falls,

→

injury, infection, excessive fatigue, and acute relapse and subsequent need for readmission to the hospital.

If the patient is not able to return home from the hospital and requires admission to another level of post-acute care, such as an SNF, the transitional care teams also need to have comprehensive communication, and the multidisciplinary rehabilitation team must be involved with the care transition. Therapists need to assess the patient's ability to physically move each joint and transfer or ambulate as well as evaluate posture, mobility, seating, wheelchair positioning, bathing, dressing, toileting, eating, swallowing function, cognition, and communication ability. Therapists also need to assess baseline and variations in vital signs such as pulse rate, respiratory rate, blood pressure, autonomic dysreflexia, pain, and arterial oxygen saturation. Their interventions throughout the stay help to promote optimal patient safety and functioning.

The ideal plan of care is very patient centered. Considerations must be made for culture, diversity of lifestyle and personal preferences, home environment, family dynamics, and natural body rhythms and routines, and all should be integrated into the plan of care created with the patient. The patient-centered approach, as well as the intensity of the therapeutic sessions, fosters trust, rapport, and the development of therapeutic relationships. The extensive observation and assessment of a patient's ongoing condition allow therapists to notice subtle warning signs or changes of condition that may be precursors to larger medical issues that would result in readmission to the hospital.

Community engagement is essential for readmission prevention. Consistent communication, collaboration, and continuity of care are needed to reduce the rate at which patients return to the hospital. Rehabilitation professionals are among the many people who play vital roles in this important discussion.

CHAPTER 12

Preventing Readmissions in Hospice and Palliative Care

The most expensive time in a Medicare beneficiary's life is the last six months before death. Hospice and palliative care partners can often be a hospital or health system's best partner in preventing unnecessary readmissions. When you consider the volume of services a patient receives under the different benefits covered by Medicare (e.g., skilled nursing, home health, hospice, palliative care), the best value is arguably provided by hospice and palliative care services. Hospice and palliative care nurses, social workers, and other team members provide daily visits and support. Other levels of care do not always allow daily visits.

Beyond delivering quality outcomes and comforting patients and family members during end-of-life care planning, preventing unnecessary hospital readmissions should be a hospice or palliative care agency's top priority. Readmission prevention is the means by which an agency sets itself apart from the others.

If they do not already have a system-owned hospice and palliative care agency, many hospitals and health systems are considering getting back into that business. Under the Affordable Care Act (ACA), the expense of not coordinating care efficiently for end-of-life patients can significantly affect an organization's ability to operate as a whole. Thus, although hospice and palliative care have not traditionally been viewed as a significant contributor to the bottom line, hospitals and health systems cannot ignore the negative consequences of not having such services in a post-ACA model.

Whether the hospice and palliative care agency is owned by the health system or is a freestanding provider, it has had to succeed in two key areas to be a preferred provider:

+ Quality
+ Patient and family satisfaction

And now, in the post-ACA era, two more key areas should be added:

+ Readmission prevention
+ Ambulatory case management (be the eyes and ears in the home, looking for risk factors)

The challenge in developing a readmission prevention strategy for hospice and palliative care is making sure staff are trained to observe for risk factors, communicate with the patient, educate the patient to self-manage, ensure patient health literacy, practice teach-back methods, and fulfill all other roles of the ambulatory case manager. For hospice and palliative care services, this extends to making sure the patient's and family's wishes are well documented and available if a patient is taken to the emergency department (ED). Knowing and understanding the patient's wishes and having the proper documentation to honor those wishes are essential.

ED physicians and staff still see the lack of documentation as a major impediment to honoring the patient's wishes. If the proper documentation is not available when a patient presents to the ED, physicians are hesitant to honor a patient's end-of-life care plan if those preferences contradict hospital policy and procedure. A hospice and palliative care agency's top priority in preventing readmissions may be summed up as follows:

The hospice and palliative care agency is responsible for ensuring that the patient and family are comfortable and that the patient does not return to the hospital unnecessarily. Further, the priority of the hospice and palliative care agency team member is to act as an ambulatory case manager by ensuring that the patient's and family's wishes are well documented and accessible to prevent unnecessary steps being taken in the ED if the patient returns to the hospital.

In short, keep the patient at home whenever possible. Health systems and insurers are not measuring hospice and palliative care agencies so much on their readmission rate as on their competency in caring for patients and not sending them to the ED unnecessarily. Thus, a hospice and palliative care provider should focus on the return-to-ED rate, not the return-to-acute-care rate.

The hospice and palliative care agency is another defensive tactic health plans can use to monitor high-risk patients in their home—and another form of ambulatory case management that does not require an investment from the health plan. Hospice and palliative care benefits often fall outside the risk responsibility of the health plan and default to the federal government.

Hospice and palliative care agencies should make sure their caretakers are trained to assess and document the same issues and risk factors that an ambulatory case manager would. Hospice and palliative care agencies that are not owned by the health system, whether part of the narrow network or not, should also train their entire team to serve in this capacity.

Hospice and palliative care agencies should use a return-to-hospital log to keep track of every patient who returns to the ED for any reason. When the agency administrator makes this a priority, discusses all return-to-ED patients every morning with the team, and shows a consistent commitment to preventing unnecessary readmissions, an agency culture of preventing unnecessary ED visits will follow.

Following are readmission prevention tactics that build on those introduced in Part II, along with a brief description of how they should be applied in a hospice and palliative care agency setting.

MAKE SURE POLST FORMS ARE AVAILABLE FOR ALL PATIENTS

Hospice and palliative care agencies must make sure that every patient has multiple copies of the Physician Orders for Life-Sustaining Treatment (POLST) form in her chart at all times. A copy of the POLST form should also be placed in a plastic sleeve and hung on or near the door in the patient's room so that if 911 emergency services are called or the patient is transported to the hospital, the paramedics can grab the plastic sleeve and take the POLST form with them to the hospital.

CONDUCT OR GAIN ACCESS TO PATIENT RISK ASSESSMENTS

Most patients referred to hospice and palliative care are considered high risk. Although hospitals are investing in risk stratification software and tools, the mere fact that a patient is referred to hospice and palliative care (in most cases for end-of-life care) suggests that he is at high risk for readmission to the hospital. It is important to understand and document the wishes and requests of the patient and family members during this challenging time. If caretakers have the proper documentation, they can communicate the patient's wishes on arrival at the ED and can back up those requests. Lack of documentation is one of the largest impediments to preventing readmissions in the hospice and palliative care area. ED physicians may provide care against the patient's wishes if they do not have the proper documentation. Hospice and palliative care agencies that know the Medicare regulations well—and ensure that proper documentation is in place and transported with the patient all times—will be successful in preventing unnecessary hospital admissions and readmissions.

PARTICIPATE IN POST-ACUTE CARE NETWORKS AND COMMUNITY COLLABORATIVES

Hospice and palliative care agencies should seek out post-acute networks or community collaboratives in their area. Although many hospitals do not include hospice and palliative care agencies in their post-acute network or community collaborative, progressive agencies will seek out those who are active in these networks and collaboratives and continue to partner with them. Hospice and palliative care agencies benefit from inclusion in the networks and collaboratives because they can stay abreast of data, current events, and requests from their major referral sources.

MAKE SURE YOU ARE PART OF THE HOSPITAL'S NARROW NETWORK

Hospice and palliative care agencies are not always included in a hospital's narrow network. If they are, that in itself is a victory. If an agency is not included in a narrow network, it should identify which skilled-nursing facilities (SNFs), home health agencies, and other providers are part of the hospital's coordinated care network so that it can continue to aggressively reach out to these facilities.

IDENTIFY LOCAL TRANSITIONAL CARE PROGRAMS

Hospice and palliative care providers should first identify which transitional care program is being used by the hospital or in the community, then read up on the specific program and make sure employees are prepared to fulfill their role in the process.

For example, several transitional care programs provide palliative care as an option. A palliative care referral is often the first step toward hospice care planning. Understanding how palliative care is handled in a transitional care program is essential for agencies to lead and innovate in the designated market.

PROVIDE AMBULATORY CASE MANAGEMENT SERVICES

While other levels of post-acute care are still learning the ropes of ambulatory case management, hospice and palliative care providers have been doing it for years. Hospice and palliative care agencies are not just caretakers but are round-the-clock case managers. By doing an effective job of case management and having proper documentation in place before an unplanned hospital visit, unnecessary readmissions can be avoided.

PROVIDE REMOTE MONITORING SERVICES

Although remote monitoring is an innovative and new technology for many post-acute care providers, it is not new in the hospice and palliative care sector. Various remote monitoring devices have been available for many years to monitor high-risk patients at end of life. Advances in technology, however, have opened the door for an increasing number of remote monitoring devices to be used for patients receiving hospice and palliative care services.

COLLECT FACILITY-SPECIFIC DATA

As with other levels of care, it is imperative that hospice and palliative care agencies understand how well they are coordinating care by collecting data. The data should be reviewed by your clinical staff and leadership team monthly and the results shared with referral sources, payers, and hospital partners. Tracking and sharing your success will show that you are a progressive and innovative agency.

CONNECT VIA A HEALTH INFORMATION EXCHANGE

All hospice and palliative care agencies should be committed to connecting electronically with their key referral partners as soon as possible. Although electronic health information exchange is not yet on the radar of many hospitals or health systems, hospitals will begin to look outward and realize the importance of connecting electronically with post-acute care providers, including hospice and palliative care agencies, that share their goal of getting the patient home.

Hospitals and health systems will start to realize that a significant portion of the reimbursement in their risk models is being spent on patients receiving hospice and palliative care and end-of-life care. As accountable care organizations become better at managing patients, hospice and palliative care and end-of-life care will become more of a focus of health information exchanges in the future.

HAVE A CONSISTENT MARKETING PLAN

Hospice and palliative care agencies can benefit from more consistent marketing and should develop a strategic and specific marketing plan that includes monthly data distribution to their referral sources. Monthly data are typically not available until around the tenth of the following month, so on the fifteenth of each month the hospice and palliative care marketer should deliver an information package to each of her key contacts.

The information package should include monthly readmission reports and remote monitoring success stories for each patient from that referral source. The package should be accompanied by a handwritten note from the marketer thanking the contact for his business and noting the marketer's availability to answer any questions. The marketer should be sure to indicate that she will be back in touch on the fifteenth of the next month with new readmission data and genetic maps.

Progressive hospice and palliative care agencies also notify the hospital when a patient is successfully transitioned home without a readmission within 30 days of the index stay. This simple action speaks volumes to your referral source. Consider celebrating the achievement by sending the hospital a congratulatory e-mail, letter, or certificate on behalf of the care coordination team with language such as the following:

> On behalf of Hometown Hospice and Palliative Care, we would like to thank you for trusting us with the care of patient F. Smith. We are writing to advise you that Ms. Smith transitioned safely home under the care of our team. It has been 30 days since she was discharged from your hospital, and we are pleased to inform you that she has not been readmitted to any hospital and continues to get stronger and recover at home. Thank you again for trusting us with the care of this patient. We appreciate your partnership and shared commitment to quality and preventing avoidable readmissions.

An innovative hospice and palliative care marketer could also send this certificate or letter (on agency letterhead, of course) to the physician's office and to the hospital case management team as a marketing tactic. Marketing in hospice and palliative care is unique, so weaving your readmission data and prevention efforts into the compassionate care you provide will become more and more essential as coordinated care networks evolve. That said, most hospice and palliative care agencies have yet to implement tactics of this nature.

TRIAGE THE PATIENT WHEN AN ACUTE CARE EPISODE OCCURS

When an acute episode occurs, it is critical that a hospice and palliative care agency take immediate action. If a patient is experiencing discomfort or pain, caretakers and operators should be trained to avoid sending him to the ED automatically unless the situation is clearly an emergency. If it is not an emergency, the agency could take the following actions:

- Refer the patient to her primary care physician's office.
- Send the patient to an urgent care clinic.
- Have the patient visit the post-acute care clinic.
- Send a home health nurse or therapist to the patient's home.
- Have the patient or caregiver contact a pharmacist to answer medication questions.
- Contact a family member to discuss ways to provide additional support and potential alternative care options.
- Transfer the patient directly to the SNF, long-term acute care hospital, or acute rehabilitation hospital if the patient was discharged from the hospital in the prior 30 days.

If the situation is not an emergency, the goal is to contact someone who can provide necessary information, help, or comfort while avoiding an unnecessary hospital readmission. Hospice and palliative care agencies should be advocates of their role in preventing unnecessary hospital readmissions.

IMPLEMENT TRANSFERS DIRECTLY FROM THE ED TO HOME WITH HOSPICE OR PALLIATIVE CARE

Discharging a patient home from the ED with an order for hospice or palliative care was rare during the fee-for-service era because this was not the most financially lucrative approach for physicians or hospitals. The "admit when we can" mentality that became common during the fee-for-service era often stifled innovative thinking and models of care that would have led to patients being discharged directly home from the ED with an order for hospice or palliative care. As hospitals and health systems adapt to the ACA, all types of transfers directly from the ED to post-acute care will become more common.

Such options might include transfers directly from the ED to an SNF or transfers to home with referral for hospice and palliative care. The new approach will require educating ED physicians and ED case managers to make sure they understand the level of services available to patients in the home and at every other level of care.

SUMMARY

As hospitals and health systems adapt to the ACA, they will begin to initiate programs that coordinate care more efficiently, focus more on the patient's wishes, and reduce unnecessary spending. Accomplishing these three goals will require health systems to develop new strategic plans. In addition to the tactics identified in this chapter, the accompanying Perspectives provide expert input on addressing readmissions in the hospice and palliative care space.

Although most people associate hospice and palliative care with end-of-life and comfort care, the last 90 days of an older person's life are often the most traumatic to his body because frequent rehospitalization is the norm. This chapter aims to provide tactics to reduce the frequency of unnecessary hospitalizations during comfort care and the end-of-life process to provide as much dignity as possible to the patient as his body shuts down physically.

Hospice and palliative care continues to be delivered by compassionate caretakers who are committed to providing as much dignity as possible to patients in their final days. In addition to keeping a focus on compassionate care, hospice and palliative care caretakers will need to add to their skill set the ability to manage patients without unnecessary hospital readmissions. The transition should be easy because these caretakers have always been patient focused, and the basic principle of these tactics is to honor the patient's wishes and have the documentation needed to back up these wishes. As hospice and palliative care caretakers refine their skills, providers will see an opportunity to increase their market share in a post-ACA era.

PERSPECTIVE
The Pharmacist's Role in Readmission Prevention: Medication Therapy Management

By Kerjun Chang, PharmD, and Sheetal Amin, PharmD, Healthy Living Pharmacy, Yorba Linda, California

Medication therapy management (MTM), especially because of the nature of the patient population to which it is targeted, is an effective way outpatient pharmacists

→

can play a role in reducing hospital readmissions. Health plans generally set certain criteria when qualifying patients as eligible for MTM services, and these criteria target patients at greatest risk for incurring high healthcare costs because of medication problems. Common criteria include advanced age, complex medication regimen, large number of medications, and such chronic disease conditions as heart failure, asthma, chronic obstructive pulmonary disease (COPD), diabetes, hypertension, and hyperlipidemia. Many of these conditions—for example, heart failure exacerbations, myocardial infarctions, and COPD exacerbations—are associated with the highest readmission rates. MTM services can improve outcomes and reduce overall healthcare costs. A large portion of the healthcare dollars saved by MTM is attributable to the prevention of hospitalizations, many of which would have been readmissions.

Many community pharmacies have already implemented MTM programs as community pharmacists take on evolving roles that are shifting from the provision of products toward the provision of clinical services. Although the provision of MTM services is still a maturing field, community pharmacists are one of the most accessible providers of clinical services for patients, so tapping the potential of pharmacist-implemented MTM will play an important role in the years ahead as efforts continue to reduce hospital readmission rates and improve patient outcomes. To that end, our pharmacy has implemented MTM programs with the aid of third-party administrators such as OutcomesMTM (www.outcomesmtm.com) and Mirixa (www.mirixa.com).

Among the challenges facing pharmacists who wish to provide MTM services are the difficulty of identifying eligible patients and getting reimbursed for their services. MTM administrators help implement MTM by contracting with

→

health plans and providing referrals for eligible patients—whether or not they are regular patients of the pharmacy—as well as streamlining the reimbursement process.

As an example of the everyday value that a community pharmacist can contribute through MTM, in our provision of MTM services using a third-party program administrator, we identified a patient with COPD who had no controller inhaler in her regimen and had been using her rescue inhaler frequently throughout the day to alleviate difficulty in breathing; she had somehow fallen off controller inhaler therapy because of coverage issues. Despite recent and multiple hospitalizations for COPD exacerbations, she did not understand the importance of the controller inhaler in reducing the risk of exacerbations. As a result of relying on her rescue inhaler, she had also experienced frequent palpitations as an adverse effect. We counseled her on the importance of the controller inhaler and contacted her physician to recommend a new prescription for a controller inhaler that was covered by insurance. As a result, we were able to restart her on controller therapy, which has been shown to reduce the risk of COPD exacerbations that require hospitalization. Additionally, the patient was also able to reduce her use of the rescue inhaler and thus experienced palpitations less frequently.

Postdischarge Medication Review and Patient Education

The hospitalization, discharge, and postdischarge periods are intense for patients and their families. During this time they have to deal with many changes, including changes to their lifestyle, medications, and daily schedule. Patient education is usually provided during the discharge period—patients and families are given directions on follow-up care, how to care for and monitor themselves, and what

→

medications to take and how to take them. In many cases, this education is done by a nurse over a short, often inadequate, amount of time. When patients are overwhelmed with information, confusion, nonadherence, and other problems may arise—underlining the importance of proper medication reconciliation, coordination of follow-up care, and patient education, which many hospitals focus on in efforts to reduce readmission rates. Although the hospital has primary responsibility for ensuring the proper provision of these aspects of care, outpatient pharmacists can act as a safety net for patients who have not received these services properly through the hospital.

For example, our pharmacy filled and delivered presecriptions for a patient who had just been discharged from a hospital. The next day, the pharmacist called the patient to provide a consultation and perform a complete review of all of his current medications. On review, multiple cases of duplicate therapy were discovered; for instance, the patient was prescribed two different forms of long-acting insulin—one of which he had been taking before hospitalization and had not been instructed to discontinue. Whether this case was an example of improper medication reconciliation or discharge counseling was not clear, the pharmacist was able to identify the issue, resolve it with the prescriber, and correctly counsel the patient to avoid duplicate therapy.

As mentioned, an important barrier to overcome in providing MTM services to patients recently discharged from the hospital is the difficulty of getting reimbursed. Although Medicare Part D supports the use of pharmacist-specific Current Procedural Terminology (CPT) codes to bill for clinical services, the relevant CPT codes require a face-to-face intervention; therefore, in the foregoing example, the pharmacist would not have been reimbursed through

→

pharmacist CPT codes. Furthermore, with Medicare Part D, any pharmacist wishing to seek reimbursement for such clinical services needs to be diligent in meeting all of the requirements to properly document the intervention. Although community pharmacists may participate in and be reimbursed for clinical services that play a role in reducing hospital readmissions, they still face barriers to reimbursement, and streamlining the reimbursement process may help to expand this role in the future.

Medication Unit Dosing as a Method for Improving Adherence
Hospitalization, especially for conditions associated with the highest readmission rates, can result in many medication changes for a patient. Multiple medications may be added to the patient's existing regimen, which is often already extensive in the case of chronic conditions associated with high rates of hospitalization and readmissions. Imagine the challenge a patient faces in taking more than ten medications daily with different directions, dosing times, and frequencies. Many patients, whether inadvertently or intentionally, become nonadherent because of the difficulty and burden of the medication regimen and are prone to medication errors. Patients with multiple medications and complex regimens can benefit from such aids as medication lists and pill boxes to simplify the task. Pharmacies can assist patients with high medication burdens by dispensing medication in unit-dosed packaging, similar to the monthly bubble-packed medications pharmacies commonly dispense to nursing facilities to reduce the risk of administration errors.

Our pharmacy, which has experience in providing medication to a number of nursing facilities, is familiar with the benefits of simplifying complex medication regimens with a high pill

$\rightarrow$

burden and different methods of unit dosing. For example, the pharmacy can package together all medications that are to be taken in a single dose and can clearly label the medication, directions, and dosing time. We have extended this service to our patients who are not being cared for in nursing homes but are having difficulty taking their medication because of pill burden. Again, reimbursement is a major barrier to providing such a service because the time and labor cost of repacking medication is not trivial, nor is the cost of the equipment and packaging material involved. However, some pharmacies may consider this service if they can provide it for a large enough number of patients or if it is feasible to charge a small fee for providing unit-dosing services to patients who may benefit from it.

Future studies comparing the outcomes of patients with high pill burdens who are provided unit-dosed medication with those who do not take unit-dosed medication would be useful in establishing the value of the practice. The expected benefits of unit dosing—increased adherence, reduced medication errors, improved outcomes, and lower overall healthcare costs—may be the compelling justification for universally reimbursing for such a service in the case of patients who can benefit from it. Technology also stands to play a vital role in expanding this service because when the appropriate robotics are no longer prohibitively expensive, the time and labor cost of providing the service would be eliminated from the equation. Along with appropriate reimbursement, the high sunk costs of implementing this type of service in high volume could easily be recouped while patients, payers, and providers reap the benefits of improved outcomes and lower healthcare costs.

PERSPECTIVE
The Role of Hospice and Palliative Care in Readmissions

By Alen Voskanian, MD
Regional medical director, VITAS Innovative Hospice Care

Palliative care, which is specialized medical care for patients with serious illness, focuses on improving quality of life by addressing pain and other symptoms. Hospice care is palliative care at the end of life that is provided by an interdisciplinary team of physicians, nurses, social workers, nurse aides, chaplains, and volunteers. Hospice provides expert medical care in addition to psychosocial and spiritual support for people facing a life-limiting illness. Hospice care is provided in multiple settings depending on where the patient resides. In most cases, hospice services are provided at the patient's home. Other settings include nursing homes, assisted-living facilities, hospitals, and freestanding hospice centers.

According to the Center to Advance Palliative Care (CAPC 2011),

> The goal of palliative care is to improve quality of life for both the patient and the family. Palliative care is provided by a team of doctors, nurses and other specialists who work with a patient's other doctors to provide an extra layer of support. Palliative care is appropriate at any age and at any stage in a serious illness, and can be provided together with curative treatment.

Healthcare Reform
The baby boomer generation started turning 65 years old in January 2011. Every day for the next 19 years, about

→

10,000 baby boomers will reach the age of 65 (Snyder 2010). This aging population will require a substantial amount of resources to address chronic medical issues and manage hospital admissions. Approximately 32 percent of total healthcare spending occurs for patients with chronic illness in their last two years of life. The sickest 5 percent of the population accounts for almost half of all healthcare expenses. Healthcare reform has focused on multiple initiatives to improve the value of medical care provided, but the following equation shows one way to assess value:

$$\text{Value of healthcare} = \frac{\text{Quality}}{\text{Cost}}$$

Before the Affordable Care Act (ACA), healthcare was volume driven and based on the fee-for-service model for reimbursement. The new initiatives generated by the ACA aim to change the focus to value-driven healthcare. One of these initiatives, the Hospital Readmission Reduction Program, is designed to improve the value equation by improving the quality of the care patients receive during hospitalization and after discharge while lowering cost. Hospital readmission rates will be used as a measure to assess improvement in care coordination and postdischarge planning.

Hospice and Readmission
When eligible terminally ill patients are referred to hospice, they are able to receive comprehensive medical care that is tailored to their needs and aligned with their goals. By addressing patients' needs proactively in a hospice setting, the need to return to the hospital is significantly reduced. Gozalo and Miller (2007) showed that nursing home residents in hospice care were less likely to be hospitalized than residents not in hospice. Furthermore, nursing home

→

residents who had a hospice informational visit had fewer acute care admissions and fewer acute care days than those who did not (mean 1.2 versus 3.0; $p = .03$) (Casarett et al. 2005). A retrospective chart review at the University of Iowa hospital showed that in the penultimate admission within 12 months of death, 60 percent of patients met National Hospice and Palliative Care Organization guidelines for hospice, and 84 percent of patients were within six months of their actual death (Freund et al. 2012). This study highlights the fact that terminally ill patients are often hospitalized multiple times as their health declines. Unfortunately, with each hospitalization, quality of life declines and patients tend to get weaker—likely because the underlying disease is progressing.

When terminally ill patients who are eligible for hospice are identified on a timely basis and referred to hospice, then the patients and families have the opportunity to benefit from the comprehensive services provided by the hospice program. Furthermore, family members become eligible to receive bereavement services. When addressed by the hospice team, patients' medical and psychosocial needs are fulfilled outside the hospital, leading to a lower readmission rate.

In conclusion, hospice and palliative care services are instrumental in improving value in the healthcare system. Hospice improves quality by managing such symptoms as pain and focusing on the goals of patients and family members. Furthermore, the care provided by the hospice team often leads to a lower rate of hospitalization and readmission, which in turn helps reduce the cost of care. Thus, better care is provided at a lower cost.

REFERENCES

Casarett, D., J. Karlawish, K. Morales, R. Crowley, T. Mirsch, and D. A. Asch. 2005. "Improving the Use of Hospice Services in Nursing Homes: A Randomized Controlled Trial." *Journal of the American Medical Association* 294 (2): 211–17.

Center to Advance Palliative Care (CAPC). 2011. *2011 Public Opinion Research on Palliative Care: A Report Based on Research by Public Opinion Strategies.* Accessed October 28, 2014. www.capc.org/tools-for-palliative-care-programs /marketing/public-opinion-research/2011-public-opinion -research-on-palliative-care.pdf.

Freund, K., M. T. Weckmann, D. J. Casarett, K. Swanson, M. K. Brooks, and A. Broderick. 2012. "Hospice Eligibility in Patients Who Died in a Tertiary Care Center." *Journal of Hospital Medicine* 7 (3): 218–23.

Gozalo, P., and S. Miller. 2007. "Hospice Enrollment and Evaluation of Its Causal Effect on Hospitalization of Dying Nursing Home Patients." *Health Services Research* 42 (2): 587–610.

Snyder, M. 2010. "In 2011 Baby Boomers Start to Turn 65: 16 Statistics About the Coming Retirement Crisis That Will Drop Your Jaw." InfoWars.com. Posted December 30. www .infowars.com/baby-boomers-start-to-turn-65-16-statistics -about-the-coming-retirement-crisis-that-will-drop-your-jaw/.

CHAPTER 13

Preventing Readmissions in Assisted-Living, Memory Care, and Board-and-Care Facilities

One factor most hospitals overlook when developing a transitional care program is identifying and partnering with leading residential facilities. As hospitals move closer to designing the delivery model of the future, however, assisted-living, memory care units, and board-and-care facilities will become a larger focus. Thus, assisted-living communities must be prepared and make readmission prevention a top priority.

Residential facilities allow patients to be cared for in a home environment. At this stage the accountable care organization (ACO), health plan, and medical group are no longer financially responsible for the expense of inpatient care. In short, patients pay their own way because rent is not considered healthcare. The health plan or payer encourages the patient to return home and provides in-home resources to aid in the rehabilitation process. The benefit is that the cost of in-home resources and services is usually 80 to 95 percent less than that for an inpatient stay.

One encouraging trend in this sector is that payers are starting to pay for more home-based services, including rent at a residential facility, as an alternative to a per diem at an inpatient facility such as a hospital or skilled-nursing facility (SNF). Such innovative thinking is the wave of the future and will largely focus on getting patients to a residential facility to reduce the costs to the payer. This is an easy sell because it is consistent with the patient's desire to return home as soon as possible.

Beyond delivering quality outcomes, achieving patient satisfaction, and ensuring profitable operations, preventing unnecessary hospital readmissions should be the top priority of an assisted-living community's executive director. Preventing readmissions is the primary means by which an assisted-living community or board-and-care facility can set itself apart from its competition. Assisted-living communities, memory care units, and board-and-care facilities must succeed in several key areas to be considered a preferred provider:

♦ Quality
♦ Patient satisfaction
♦ Physician alignment
♦ Communication with providers

And now, in the post–Affordable Care Act (ACA) era, one more key area should be added:

♦ Readmission prevention (to the acute care hospital and all other levels of care)

The executive director's challenge in developing a readmission prevention strategy for his residential community is making sure staff are trained to handle and care for as many clinical needs and situations as possible. An executive director or board-and-care owner's top priority in readmission prevention may be summed up as follows:

An assisted-living community, memory care unit, or board-and-care home is responsible for providing the necessary level of care and preventing the need for the patient to leave the facility to return to a hospital or other level of care.

Hospitals are not measuring residential communities so much on their readmission rate as on their competency in caring for patients and not sending them to the emergency department (ED) unnecessarily. Thus, a residential care facility operator should focus on the return-to-ED rate, not the return-to-acute-care rate.

Just as in an SNF, tools such as the INTERACT (Interventions to Reduce Acute Care Transfers) protocols are invaluable because they give step-by-step directions for nurses to follow when a patient's status declines. In the fee-for-service model, when a patient started to decline, an assisted-living facility nurse or caretaker would tell the physician, and the physician's response was to send the patient to the ED. In the fee-for-service model, the physician, the hospital, and potentially the SNF benefited financially each time a patient was readmitted to the hospital.

In a post-ACA environment, ACOs and health plans will aggressively attempt to avoid the SNF altogether and will call on residential communities to provide a higher level of care as an alternative to SNF days. The assisted-living sector is ready to step up and provide this higher level of care and has so far been doing so with great enthusiasm. One need not look any further than the effective programs being operated at Silverado Senior Living and Belmont Village communities nationwide. Although both of these assisted-living organizations focus on memory care, each has developed a comprehensive program with extensive clinical interventions and a nurse-to-patient ratio that is higher than the state minimum requirement for SNFs. Organizations like these demonstrate a commitment to quality care at the highest level.

Following are readmission prevention tactics that build on those introduced in Part II, along with a brief description of how they should be applied in a residential care setting.

MAKE SURE POLST FORMS ARE AVAILABLE FOR ALL PATIENTS

Assisted-living, memory care, and board-and-care leadership must make sure every patient has a Physician Orders for Life-Sustaining Treatment (POLST) form in her chart at the nursing station. A copy of the POLST form should also be placed in a plastic sleeve and hung on or near the door in the patient's room so that if 911 emergency services are called or the patient is transported to the hospital, the paramedics can grab the plastic sleeve and take the POLST form with them to the hospital.

Nurses should always send a copy of the POLST form when the patient transfers to the hospital. For this reason, three copies of the POLST form should be inside the chart at all times because the hospital rarely sends it back when the patient returns to the residential care facility.

If the executive director of an assisted-living community or a group home owner wants to set the facility apart from the competition in ways beyond superior quality, ensuring that a POLST form is sent each time a patient goes to the hospital is an ideal tactic. Almost every facility talks about doing it and claims it is done consistently, but in fact most residential care facilities do not send a POLST form every time a patient leaves the facility. This is a simple step that can go a long way toward setting a facility apart as a preferred provider.

CONDUCT OR GAIN ACCESS TO PATIENT RISK ASSESSMENTS

Although most risk stratification will take place in the acute care hospital setting, the long-term goal of coordinated care is to keep patients in their home environment. Thus, the residential care facility and its staff play an active role in obtaining a more comprehensive risk assessment of the patient. A risk assessment strategy that relies only on data gathered in the acute care setting is incomplete, though at present it is the most common form of risk stratification.

An assisted-living community that wants to set itself apart from its competitors should work with its acute care providers, health plans, and payers to find out how it can contribute to a patient's risk assessment, reminding them that the ultimate goal for everyone is to keep the patient at home. To achieve that goal, information needs to be gathered about the patient outside the acute care setting, too. In fact, the residential care facility is best positioned over the long term to provide the most pertinent and relevant information to keep the patient from being readmitted to the hospital unnecessarily.

All staff at the residential care facility should be educated on the importance of risk stratification and how to identify and communicate risk factors when they arise. One of the best tactics a residential care facility can deploy to prevent unnecessary readmissions is to use INTERACT tools and educate all staff on the steps and protocols to take when they note risk factors or see signs that a patient is deteriorating. The caretaker should rely on his experience and knowledge and on the tools the residential care facility operator has provided rather than immediately calling the physician, as was the practice in the fee-for-service model. Staff should be aware that the goal is to avoid hospitalization, and if they call the physician without specific details, the patient will almost certainly be transferred to the hospital.

The residential care facility needs to gain access to the risk tool used by the hospital or health plan. Then, when a high-risk patient arrives at the residential care facility, the staff should obtain the patient's care plan from the hospital or health plan. The facility should have a protocol to raise awareness among facility staff when a patient is at high risk for hospital readmission. The staff's goal should be to avoid hospitalization if at all possible. If leadership makes it a priority, staff will follow.

PARTICIPATE IN POST-ACUTE CARE NETWORKS AND COMMUNITY COLLABORATIVES

All residential care facility operators should seek out post-acute care networks and community collaboratives in their area. The meeting topics are not nearly as important as your presence. When a facility does not show up to the meeting, it sends a message to the hospital that readmissions are not a priority and the hospital is not an important referral source.

The biggest challenge in joining a post-acute care network or community collaborative is that many hospitals will not include residential care facilities. Hospitals that are privately owned and do not have a dedicated staff member focused on population management and coordinated care will likely limit participation to skilled nursing and home health and may not include additional levels of care.

Assisted-living facilities should be persistent in asking to attend meetings even if invitations are not typically extended to assisted-living communities. Many hospital directors find it difficult to say no, especially when the question is asked in person. For your facility to play a role in the coordinated care network, you have to be present at the meetings.

MAKE SURE YOU ARE PART OF THE HOSPITAL'S NARROW NETWORK

Assisted-living communities and group homes must position themselves and lobby to be included in any narrow network. Hospitals are narrowing their networks, and instead of referring to all of the residential care facilities in their region, they now refer to only a few preferred providers. Although many hospitals do not include assisted-living communities and board-and-care facilities in the process, as population health management becomes more of a focus in the future, hospitals will recognize that residential facilities are a key component in developing a successful coordinated care model.

Be sure to do a SWOT (strengths, weaknesses, opportunities, threats) analysis to identify weaknesses that may prevent your facility from being included in a narrow network. Consider proximity, for example. Is your facility in a hospital's 911 zone? Are you closer to another hospital? Proximity is often the top factor a hospital considers when deciding whether to include you in its narrow network. Hospitals do not want to send their patients to a post-acute care or residential facility in an area where the paramedics would be required to take 911 patients to another hospital. Do not underestimate proximity as a deciding factor for hospitals.

The other key factor that will position a residential care facility for inclusion in a narrow network is the alignment of physicians servicing the residential care facility who also work directly with the hospital. Without an active physician from the hospital who can champion your residential care facility as a quality provider that should be included in the narrow network, operators will find it difficult to get the hospital and its leaders to even engage in this conversation. Once again, be persistent in your pursuit to be included in the narrow network.

All of these factors should still be considered if it is the health plan or insurer that is narrowing the network. Understand the goals of the narrow network and who is driving it, and work relentlessly to be included.

IDENTIFY LOCAL TRANSITIONAL CARE PROGRAMS

Assisted-living operators should first identify which transitional care program is being used by the hospital or in the community. The individual tactics used by the hospital or health system to support the transitional care program are relevant to the residential care facility.

For example, several transitional care programs require a post-acute care follow-up visit to a primary care physician or high-risk patient clinic. Some hospitals are asking the residential care facility to schedule that appointment after discharge from the hospital or SNF. Residential care facilities are under no obligation to do so, but complying with the request is a good way to stay in the hospital's favor.

PROVIDE AMBULATORY CASE MANAGEMENT SERVICES

Ambulatory case management refers to the task of monitoring, servicing, and assisting the patient beyond discharge from the hospital to an SNF. One of the benefits of narrowing the home health network is that it can manage the process on behalf of the hospital and SNF. The assisted-living facility and board-and-care home can fulfill the same role.

Understanding the hospital's care plan for high-risk patients once they leave the acute care setting is critical for all assisted-living and board-and-care facilities. In the assisted-living or board-and-care environment, ambulatory case managers hired or assigned by the hospital or health plan are not necessary if the residential care facility has trained its staff to be on the alert for warning signs, to educate patients properly, and to understand the goals of value-based care and keeping patients out of the hospital when appropriate.

PROVIDE REMOTE MONITORING SERVICES

A great way for assisted-living communities and board-and-care homes to set themselves apart from their competition is to partner with a hospital and physician to provide remote monitoring services. In many states, Medicare is now reimbursing for remote monitoring devices. On discharge from the hospital, physicians can prescribe one of many different monitoring devices that will shorten hospital length of stay and allow a patient to return home sooner.

Many physicians have found that by discharging a patient to an assisted-living community or board-and-care home that has round-the-clock caretakers, their perceived liability is much less than if they discharge the patient home. Providing remote monitoring services requires only a minimal investment from the assisted-living community or board-and-care home.

The remote monitoring process is simple. The remote device is applied to the patient in the hospital or physician's office and remains in place while the patient is staying at a residential care facility. The monitoring is usually done at a central location, where the patient's vital signs are relayed via wireless technology to a data center that knows the patient's location and has a direct telephone number to the residential care facility. If the patient's remote monitoring device alerts the command center of a change in vital signs, the data center immediately notifies the facility about the changing condition.

COLLECT FACILITY-SPECIFIC DATA

All residential care facilities should examine their readmission rate monthly. A number of available software programs generate a monthly report of all patients who were readmitted to the hospital unnecessarily, and predictive software allows early identification of patients who are declining and therefore at higher risk of needing acute care. These data should be reviewed by your clinical staff and leadership team daily and shared with your hospital partners monthly. Even when hospital partners collect this information themselves, it is typically at least 12 months old because reporting mechanisms are not that advanced.

CONNECT VIA A HEALTH INFORMATION EXCHANGE

All assisted-living communities, memory care facilities, and board-and-care homes should be committed to connecting electronically with their key referral partners and start pursuing that goal as soon as possible. Although hospitals and health systems will likely not wish to connect with residential care facilities electronically for several years, it is important that residential care facility operators initiate this conversation with hospitals and health systems now. The ACA's meaningful use programs incentivize hospitals to implement electronic health records and connect with physicians via a health information exchange (HIE). Now that all of the incentives and deadlines to connect with physicians have passed, hospitals will begin to look outward and realize the importance of connecting with their post-acute and residential care providers.

HAVE A CONSISTENT MARKETING PLAN

Perhaps the most important tactic in preventing readmissions is telling your story. One of the biggest flaws in today's post-acute care model is the lack of consistent marketing from post-acute care providers, including residential care facilities. Although assisted-living communities and board-and-care facilities often undertake aggressive marketing efforts, that same focus on strategic marketing is missing in the residential care facility space.

Thus, assisted-living communities should have a strategic and specific marketing plan that showcases their focus on the tactics discussed in this chapter. Monthly data are typically not available until around the tenth of the following month, so on the fifteenth of each month the assisted-living community or board-and-care marketer should deliver an information package to each of her key contacts at the hospital.

The information package should include monthly readmission reports, remote monitoring success stories, and genetic test results and case summaries for each patient from that referral source in the prior month. The package should be accompanied by a handwritten note from the marketer thanking the contact for his business and noting the marketer's availability to answer any questions. The marketer should be sure to indicate in the note or orally that she will be back in touch on the fifteenth of the next month with new data and test results. The practice should be repeated each month until a consistent pattern is developed and the hospital begins to rely on the residential care facility and the data it provides each month.

PROMOTE SELF-MANAGEMENT, PATIENT HEALTH LITERACY, AND USE OF TEACH-BACK METHODS

Patient self-management is the most critical way to prevent readmissions at every level of care. Every residential care facility operator should make sure that staff—particularly the director of nursing, nurses, nurse aides, social workers, therapists, and discharge planners—are all committed to educating patients to care for themselves.

After all, the ultimate goal is to get the patient home safely, and the post-acute care provider's challenge is to understand the patient's home environment. Although patients are provided with caretakers in residential care facilities, that does not change the fact that all patients need to learn to care for themselves and minimize risk factors, or else hospital readmission is inevitable.

Teach-back is the methodology most commonly used to ensure patient health literacy. In this patient-education method, the patient is provided with collateral material illustrating what she has learned and is then asked to confirm comprehension by reciting back or demonstrating the protocols she needs to self-administer her care. The assisted-living community should not underestimate its role in the teach-back process.

PURSUE CONTRACT ALIGNMENT

The ACA has placed an even greater emphasis on coordinating care between providers. A coordinated care model is much like a traditional health maintenance organization in that preferred providers are included in the network. Providers should go to great lengths to keep patients within the network when they need a different level of care to ensure efficiency in a value-based care delivery model. Thus, all assisted-living communities and board-and-care homes should make sure staff are aware of their facility's primary referral hospitals, key contract partners, and post-acute care providers. One slip-up, where a residential care facility sends its patient to the wrong hospital, even in an emergency, can cause great harm with these referral sources. Although residential care facilities have never paid much attention to medical group, health plan, and insurance coverage issues, it is more important than ever that the leaders of residential care facilities and all of their care delivery staff know their primary contracting partners.

CONDUCT GENETIC TESTING

Assisted-living communities and board-and-care homes have begun to conduct genetic testing to better understand how their patients react to various medications. Not only does this allow them to better manage their patients' medication regimens, but it also reduces medication errors and lowers the overall medication cost to the residential care facility.

The procedure, which is covered by Medicare Part B as of January 1, 2014, may be conducted once in a patient's lifetime. The hospital community has been slow to order genetic maps because the benefit is not approved under Medicare Part A and hospitals are not reimbursed for inpatients. Many residential care facilities, however, recognize that genetic testing not only is a means to improve patient care but also gives them a marketing edge over their competitors. Thus, they have begun ordering these tests for their patients and sharing results with the referring hospital. The hospital, in turn, with the proper patient consent, can scan the results into the electronic health record for permanent use via the HIE. (Exhibit 9.1 in Chapter 9 shows a sample genetic testing report.)

NARROW THE HOME HEALTH NETWORK AND COORDINATE HOME HEALTH SERVICES

It is critical that assisted-living communities and group homes know which home health agencies are used by their key referring hospitals. In fact, if a residential care facility is acting in the best interest of the patient and the coordinated care model, it would stop referring to all home health agencies other than those used by the hospital from which the patient was transferred.

This can cause a conundrum for assisted-living facilities because they often have their own integrated programs for home health and therapy services. Historically, when a patient was discharged from an assisted-living facility with an order for a home health evaluation, the assisted-living facility usually rejected the order or honored it but provided its own level of service. This decision may have been financially motivated, or it may have been made because the assisted-living community had its own internal coordinated care program. Whatever the reason, these types of programs put the facility's position as a preferred provider at risk. In contrast, in a post-ACA environment, the hospital and health system seek post-acute care partners that are completely committed to their coordinated care model.

In other words, referral partners do not want to work with post-acute care facilities or assisted-living communities that pick and choose which parts of the coordinated care model they will honor. In short, if an assisted-living facility has its own home health or therapeutic program that it views as a replacement for the network's designated home health care provider or providers, it should consider using the network provider for all patients referred within the network as a means to honor its acute referral partner.

ADOPT INTERACT TOOLS

INTERACT offers several free tools that have been developed for assisted-living communities and group home operators to implement in their facility to improve their ability to coordinate care with acute providers (see http://interact2.net). If a residential care facility has not implemented these tools, it risks being excluded from a hospital's list of preferred providers, narrow network, and transitional care program. At a minimum, all residential care facilities should review and consider implementing these tools to prevent unnecessary readmissions to the hospital.

INVEST IN PREDICTIVE SOFTWARE

Residential care facilities that are committed to preventing unnecessary hospital readmissions and coordinating care with referral partners invest in predictive software. The software provides early identification of a patient who is declining, alerts the care team, and provides a pathway and recommendations on how best to stabilize the patient so that a hospital readmission is avoided.

Although many skilled-nursing and assisted-living communities use the INTERACT protocols, which continue to innovate and become more electronically integrated, such tools are retrospective and focus on educating staff after a readmission has occurred. In contrast, predictive software prevents the readmission. Predictive software is available for assisted-living facilities and should be considered by any assisted-living community, memory care unit, or board-and-care facility that wants to show its hospital referral partners that it seeks to be the preferred provider for residential care services. Exhibit 3.1 (in Chapter 3) shows a sample predictive software report.

IMPLEMENT DIRECT-FROM-ED AND OBSERVATION UNIT TRANSFERS

Hospitals and health systems are slowly moving toward a model in which they will more aggressively discharge patients directly from the ED to post-acute care in residential care facilities. At present, this type of discharge can be difficult because the financial pieces often take several days to coordinate. However, progressive assisted-living communities and board-and-care homes will seek out their hospital or health system partner to propose a rapid-discharge agreement that allows the hospital to get patients to the residential care facility without delay.

The residential care facility could propose one of several financial arrangements to the hospital or health system. These arrangements range from a risk-sharing agreement, for patients who are not able to pay for the stay, to a bed-lease arrangement, where the hospital reimburses the assisted-living community or board-and-care home for total days at the end of each month. The financial arrangement will be driven by what the hospital is willing to commit to.

When I meet with hospital C-suite executives to discuss this tactic, I suggest starting with a proposal to create a partnership for same-day discharge for patients with no payer source. The partnership would cover situations where it takes a few days to confirm a patient's insurance coverage or financial arrangements. This arrangement would help hospitalists meet their goal of minimizing length of stay and ensure improved patient flow in the hospital. The residential care facility may also want to commit to having a social worker and discharge planner who will seek permanent placement for patients once they arrive at the facility. Hospitals would consider this a valuable service. The tactic is not widely used at present but will become more prevalent as assisted-living communities and board-and-care homes are able to tell the hospital C-suite about the opportunity.

SUMMARY

It will likely be a few years before assisted-living communities and board-and-care homes become the primary source of hospital and ED discharges, but that day will come as a result of the ACA. Just as with post-acute care providers, residential care facilities must go to great lengths to pay attention to preventing unnecessary readmissions. By using the tactics described in this chapter and its accompanying Perspective, an assisted-living community, memory care facility, or board-and-care home will be well positioned to become a preferred provider with each of its referral sources.

Once your facility team has considered, reviewed, discussed, and implemented these tactics, your marketing staff should tell your story by providing a comprehensive data packet to referral sources on a monthly basis. Once these tactics have been mastered, facility leaders can begin educating caretakers and physicians who visit the assisted-living community or board-and-care facility about the value-added programs and solutions the facility provides. At that point, the community will be well aware that your assisted-living community or board-and-care home is a high-quality service provider and a preferred provider for all local referral sources.

PERSPECTIVE
Helping Patients and Their Caregivers Find Hope in Realistic Healthcare Goals

By Nicholas Jauregui, MD
Palliative care medical director, Huntington Hospital
Pasadena, California

The key to significantly reducing preventable readmissions to hospitals is found not in new expensive technology and programs but in a better understanding of the human person in the context of the patient's family, caregivers, and support community. The answer to the hospital readmission problem is found in a wellness approach to care and not merely in disease modification.

The current healthcare system focuses on treating illness and specializes in organ systems. In the usual care of patients, healthcare providers rarely focus on asking the patient and his family what they are hoping to accomplish with healthcare.

When we do ask the patient and family what they are hoping for or what the goals of medical care are for the patient in the context of her caregivers, we often fail to ask if their hopes and goals are realistically achievable with the current medical technology. Most important, our healthcare system rarely guides the patient and family to find hope in realistic goals for medical care.

Even with the most advanced medical technology in the hands of the best and most experienced clinicians, we will have to help many patients—and eventually all patients— face the reality that disease-modifying care has reached its limit. When this limit is reached and we treat a patient in the hospital and discharge him without making sure he, →

his family, and other caregivers realize that his condition will further decline despite the best treatments, we have set ourselves up for a readmission in the near future.

Such a readmission cannot be prevented with better medical treatment designed to monitor and modify the disease. The only medical care that will prevent this readmission will be guiding the patient, family, and other relevant caregivers to find hope in a realistic medical care plan that does not include a readmission to the hospital but rather care in the home setting or another setting in the post-acute care continuum.

Most often, the community resources available to help the patient and family in their home setting at no cost to the hospital are not used sufficiently. Guiding the patient, family, and other caregivers to find hope in a realistic and medically achievable care plan is generally achieved in a family meeting with a physician or nurse practitioner who is familiar with the medical conditions affecting the patient. The clinician must have within her scope of practice the ability to diagnose illness and explain the intimate details of all aspects of the patient's illness. Patients, families, and caregivers cannot find hope in realistic goals for medical care if they do not sufficiently understand all of the serious illnesses involved. These family meetings may require one hour or more to achieve a good outcome.

A well-trained physician or nurse practitioner will be able to guide the patient, family, and other caregivers to a care plan that is realistic and often achievable at home rather than the acute care setting when disease-modifying treatments are no longer able to rehabilitate the patient. The family meeting must be positive and focused on what can be done to

→

improve the quality of life for the patient and family and not on what cannot be accomplished with the current disease-modifying technology. Presenting the options of comfort-focused care in the home when that is medically appropriate is too often not presented as a hope-filled option to patients and their families.

Our goal as healthcare providers should be to add value to the care of the patient and family through these family meetings and thus improve the quality of care, enhance the patient and family's experience with care, and reduce avoidable readmissions. The goals of a good supportive-care family meeting should be threefold:

1. Guide patients and their families to meet their highest potential health and develop a medical care plan in which they find hope in realistic goals for the patient's medical care.
2. Manage symptoms and coordinate and assist in healthcare planning across care transitions.
3. Help patients, their families, referring physicians, and other caregivers experience how wellness and sup-portive care have a unique and positive effect on a patient's care plan that results in high satisfaction.

On discharge, the patient and family need to have care brought to them in the home setting so that they do not have to tough it out until they see their doctor or become so desperate that they return to the emergency department—and then, all too often, are readmitted to the hospital.

The supportive-care family meeting should take a wellness approach that puts in place a home support system for the patient and family, often through a supportive-care program

$\rightarrow$

arranged by a home health agency in collaboration with a supportive-care specialty medical group, where the focus is on helping the patient and family meet their highest potential quality of life. This is true wellness in the context of a patient with a serious disease. In this framework of supportive care we can develop highly effective transitional care programs, palliative care programs, and hospice programs. The focus of care becomes hope in wellness and quality of life despite the patient's serious illness.

Care of this type integrates the physical, social, psychological, and spiritual needs of the patient, in contrast to the problem-focused and often organ-focused healthcare that generally reacts to problems and all too often only does so in the emergency department, resulting in avoidable readmissions. The key to stopping readmissions is found in helping the patient, family, and caregivers find hope in realistic goals for their medical care.

CHAPTER 14

Preventing Readmissions in Home Care and Private-Duty Nursing

If all health systems seek to discharge patients home as the first alternative from all levels of care, then home health services are certain to grow. If home health services (which are covered by Medicare) see explosive growth in coming years, then nonmedical home care and private-duty nursing services will also see explosive growth. This is especially true if hospitals and health systems own and manage their own home health agency.

Home care and *private-duty nursing* are the terms typically used to describe the in-home support services provided to patients once they are discharged from medical and therapy-based home health services (funded for Medicare and commercial payers). All patients who are discharged from home health services should be given an order for home care or private-duty nursing because it acts as a bridge from the inpatient setting to the home setting and provides oversight for a patient's care in her everyday setting.

Home care and private-duty nursing are privately paid benefits; they are not paid for by the insurer. Therefore, it is in the best interests of the hospital and payer not only to discharge all patients to home health after an emergency department (ED) visit, acute care stay, or skilled-nursing stay but also to order home care once home health services are completed.

Ideally, home care should happen automatically and should be viewed as another form of ambulatory case management and an added resource for patients and their families. In fact, even when a patient who comes to the ED does not need home health services, physicians may recommend a caretaker, home care, or a private-duty nurse for additional support.

Patient choice and antisteering regulations are not as relevant an issue when the services are not reimbursed by the federal government, as is the case with home care and private-duty nursing services. Simply stated, home health agencies are required to offer patients a choice because they are Medicare participants, but they have more leeway when dealing with services such as home care and private-duty nursing, which are not reimbursed by the Medicare benefit.

A health system–owned home health agency should make sure its caretakers are trained to assess and document the same clinical issues and risk factors that an ambulatory case manager would if sent into the home environment. Home health agencies that are not owned by the health system, whether part of its narrow network or not, should also train their entire team to serve in this capacity. This same approach should be extended into home care and private-duty nursing services.

The home care and private-duty caretaker model has been attempted in many variations by commercial health plans. Although the model has room for improvement, caretakers at all points of care now start their patient evaluation with one basic question: Can we discharge this patient home safely and confidently? This type of model plays well in a home health, home care, and private duty–based system.

With the understanding that growth in the home care or private-duty nursing sector is inevitable, a home health provider must succeed in several key areas to become a preferred provider:

- Quality
- Patient satisfaction
- Ease of referral and discharge process
- Response-to-referral times
- Efficient communication systems

And now, in the post–Affordable Care Act (ACA) era, two more key areas should be added:

- 30-day readmission prevention systems
- Ambulatory case management (act as the eyes and ears in the home, looking for risk factors)

The challenge for home care and private-duty nursing when developing a readmission prevention strategy is making sure all staff members are trained to watch for risk factors, communicate with the patient, prepare the patient to self-manage, ensure patient health literacy, practice teach-back methods, and fulfill all other roles of the ambulatory case manager. The top priority for a home care and private-duty nursing agency in readmission prevention may be summed up as follows:

> Home care and private-duty nursing agencies are responsible for ensuring that the patient continues to rehabilitate at home and does not return to the hospital unnecessarily. Further, the home care team member's priority is to act as an ambulatory case manager by ensuring that the home is safe and free of risk factors.

In short, keep the patient at home whenever possible. Health systems and insurers are not measuring home care agencies so much on their readmission rate as on their competency in caring for patients and not sending them to the ED unnecessarily. Thus, a health agency provider should focus on the return-to-ED rate, not the return-to-acute-care rate.

Much like home health agencies, home care and private-duty nursing agencies should use a return-to-hospital log and keep track of every patient who returns to the ED for any reason. When the agency administrator makes this a priority, discusses all return-to-ED patients every morning with the home care team, and shows a consistent commitment to preventing unnecessary readmissions, an agency culture of preventing unnecessary ED visits will follow.

Following are readmission prevention tactics that build on those introduced in Part II, along with a brief description of how they should be applied in a home care agency setting.

MAKE SURE POLST FORMS ARE AVAILABLE FOR ALL PATIENTS

Home care agencies must make sure that every patient has a Physician Orders for Life-Sustaining Treatment (POLST) form. A copy of the POLST form should also be placed in a plastic sleeve and hung on or near the door of the patient's home so it is in the line of sight for paramedics and other key point people. If 911 emergency services are called or the patient is transported to the hospital, the paramedics can grab the plastic sleeve and take the POLST form with them to the hospital.

Nurses should always send a copy of the POLST form when the patient transfers to the hospital. For this reason, three copies of the POLST form should be available at all times because the hospital rarely sends it back home with the patient.

CONDUCT OR GAIN ACCESS TO PATIENT RISK ASSESSMENTS

The home care agency and private-duty nursing staff should be made aware of high-risk patients. They also need to understand the health system or payer's plan for each high-risk patient. Some coordination, planning, and aligned software packages may be required for home care agencies to adequately support the health system's plan for these specific patients. However, home care agencies that are progressive and hope to thrive in a post-ACA era should make sure they can support the protocols that health plans, health systems, and hospitals use to prevent high-risk patients from being readmitted to the hospital.

PARTICIPATE IN POST-ACUTE CARE NETWORKS AND COMMUNITY COLLABORATIVES

Home care agencies should seek out post-acute care networks or community collaboratives in their area. The topics of meetings are not nearly as important as your presence there. When a home care agency does not show up at the meeting, it sends a message to the hospital that readmissions are not a priority and the hospital is not important as a referral source. Progressive home care agencies that make these collaboratives a priority and support them in whatever capacity possible will be better positioned to succeed in a post-ACA era.

If the hospitals that refer to you do not have their own post-acute care network and there is no community collaborative, consider taking the lead in partnering with the home health agency of choice (the one that is aligned with the high-volume discharging hospital) in forming a community collaborative. If the hospital limits its post-acute care network to skilled-nursing facilities (SNFs), make sure you know which facilities those are so that you can focus your marketing efforts on them. Home care agencies should also know which home health agencies are in the narrow network.

MAKE SURE YOU ARE PART OF THE
HOSPITAL'S NARROW NETWORK

Although home care agencies have not traditionally been considered part of a coordinated care network, this trend will change in coming years, so home care agencies must position themselves and lobby to be included in any narrow network. Hospitals are narrowing their networks, and rather than referring to all of the home care agencies in their region, they may refer to only a few preferred providers.

Although many health systems consider home care and private-duty nursing agencies an extension beyond post-acute care into privately provided services, some of the more progressive health systems have begun to emphasize the importance of home care and private-duty nursing. Progressive home care agencies should lobby their local hospital, health system, and health plan to move in this direction.

In communities where the idea of home care agencies being included in the care network is still in the distant future, progressive home care agencies should seek out the identified post-acute care providers in the coordinated care network. For example, a home care agency should know which SNFs and home health agencies are preferred providers and which are not. In a sense, a home care agency can informally insert itself into the coordinated care network by aligning with post-acute care providers that are aligned with the acute care hospital.

IDENTIFY LOCAL TRANSITIONAL
CARE PROGRAMS

Home care providers should first identify which transitional care program is being used by the hospital or in the community, then read up on the specific program and make sure employees are pre-pared to fulfill their role in the process.

For example, several transitional care programs require a post-acute care follow-up visit to a primary care physician or high-risk patient clinic. Some health systems have started asking the home care agency or private-duty nurse to serve as an ambulatory case manager and schedule the follow-up appointment after discharge from the hospital or SNF. Home care agencies are under no obligation to do so, but complying with the request is a way to stay in the hospital's good graces.

PROVIDE AMBULATORY CASE MANAGEMENT SERVICES

Ambulatory case management refers to the task of monitoring, servicing, and assisting the patient beyond discharge from the hospital to an SNF. One of the benefits of narrowing the home health network is that the home care team can manage this process on behalf of the hospital and SNF.

The main goals of an ambulatory case management home visit are to

- confirm that the patient has safely transferred to his living environment,
- ensure that the patient understands his medication regimen and has an adequate supply of medication,
- ensure that the patient is comfortable and not anxious about self-management or his living environment, and
- identify risk factors in the home environment visually on a visit or through questions on a phone call.

The home care service provider is an ideal caretaker to fulfill this role, and this will likely be the most critical factor health systems and payers consider when choosing their preferred home care providers. Thus, it is important that a home care agency and its staff be willing to spend a few extra minutes doing ambulatory case management on behalf of the payer.

Another way to make your home care and private-duty agency stand out from the others is to implement a process for notifying hospitals and primary care physicians as a courtesy when a patient is discharged from the SNF to home, specifically patients within the 30-day discharge window (often, the physician is unaware that a hospitalist and SNF handled the patient). An agency might consider taking it a step further by including in the hospital notification a plan to update the hospital on the patient's 72-hour post-discharge visit and then again a week later. Doing so will position your agency as a preferred provider over the competition.

PROVIDE REMOTE MONITORING SERVICES

A great way for home care agencies to distinguish themselves from their competition is to partner with a hospital and physician to support remote monitoring services. In many states, Medicare is now reimbursing for remote monitoring devices. When discharging a patient from the hospital, physicians can prescribe one of many different monitoring devices that will shorten hospital length of stay and allow a patient to return home sooner.

COLLECT AGENCY-SPECIFIC DATA

As with other levels of care, home care agencies must understand how well they are coordinating care by collecting data. The data should be reviewed by your clinical staff and leadership team monthly and the results shared with referral sources, payers, and hospital partners. Tracking and sharing your success will show that you are a progressive and innovative provider.

CONNECT VIA A HEALTH INFORMATION EXCHANGE

All home care agencies should be committed to connecting electronically with their key referral partners as soon as possible. Although this is not yet on the radar of many hospitals and health systems, hospitals will soon begin to look outward and realize the importance of connecting with their post-acute care providers, including the privately funded home care and private-duty nursing agencies that share their goal of getting the patient home.

Hospitals and health systems will also realize that the handoff from home health services to home care or private-duty nursing is a symbolic transition from post-acute care to a healthy lifestyle or wellness. As hospitals move beyond the fee-for-service era and see that the ACA is designed to incentivize healthy lifestyles and wellness, initiatives such as connecting electronically with home-based providers will become more of a priority.

HAVE A CONSISTENT MARKETING PLAN

Home care agencies can benefit from more consistent marketing to referral sources and should develop a strategic and specific marketing plan that includes monthly data distribution to their referral sources. Monthly data are typically not available until around the tenth of the following month, so on the fifteenth of each month the home health marketer should deliver an information package to each of her key contacts at the hospital and SNF. This information package should include monthly readmission reports and remote monitoring success stories for each patient referred from that source in the prior month.

The package should be accompanied by a handwritten note from the marketer thanking the contact for his business and noting the marketer's availability to answer any questions. The marketer should be sure to indicate that she will be back in touch on the fifteenth of the next month with new data. Consistency in delivering this information speaks volumes to referral sources.

Marketing efforts to referral sources should target hospital inpatient units, observation units, and the ED. Primary care physicians' offices, high-risk clinics, SNFs, home health agencies, and all other post-acute care providers should also be targeted.

Progressive home care agencies also notify the hospital when a patient is successfully transitioned home without a readmission within 30 days of the index stay. This simple action demonstrates your commitment in partnering with your referral source. Consider celebrating this achievement by sending the hospital a congratulatory e-mail, letter, or certificate on behalf of the care coordination team with language such as the following:

> On behalf of the Hometown Home Care Agency, we would like to thank you for trusting us with the care of patient F. Smith. We are writing to advise you that Mr. Smith transitioned home safely under the care of our home care team. It has been 30 days since he was discharged from your hospital, and we are pleased to inform you that he has not been readmitted to any hospital. Thank you again for trusting us with the care of this patient. We appreciate your partnership and shared commitment to quality and preventing avoidable readmissions.

The home care marketer could also send this certificate or letter (on agency letterhead, of course), to the physician's office and to the hospital case management team as a marketing tactic.

PROMOTE SELF-MANAGEMENT, PATIENT HEALTH LITERACY, AND USE OF TEACH-BACK METHODS

Patient self-management is the most critical way to prevent readmissions at every level of care. Every home care agency's goal should be to make sure that all staff are committed to educating patients to care for themselves. Although this may seem to contradict its overall business goal, an agency that is committed to patients' well-being and quality of life should be focused on teaching them to manage their own care.

A patient must have a clear understanding of how to best care for her individual needs. The home-based caretaker is in the ideal position to identify the challenges and risk factors in the patient's home environment to help her identify a care plan to overcome the most significant challenges. This may be as simple as helping the patient climb the stairs on her own, helping her understand how to take her medications, or ensuring that there is enough nutritious food in the refrigerator to last through the week. Whatever the task, the home care agency and private-duty nurse are well positioned to play an important role in using teach-back methods and ensuring patient self-management.

The home care agency caretaker should never underestimate his role in this process. If the home care agency hopes to be included in a narrow network and be viewed as a preferred provider, it must take an active, calculated role in fulfilling the educational mission of the transitional care program, post-acute care network, or community collaborative.

PURSUE CONTRACT ALIGNMENT

Health plans have started to include private-duty nursing and home care as a provided or reimbursable service. Thus, progressive home care agencies should seek out these health plans and insurers to make sure they are included as a contracted provider when the payer is prepared to have this discussion.

TRIAGE THE PATIENT WHEN AN ACUTE CARE EPISODE OCCURS

When an acute episode occurs, it is essential that the home care agency take immediate action to avoid a readmission. Thus, when a patient calls because he is experiencing discomfort or pain, caretakers and operators should be trained to avoid sending him to the ED automatically unless the situation is an emergency only the ED is capable of managing. If it is not an emergency, the agency could take the following actions:

- Refer the patient to his primary care physician's office.
- Send the patient to an urgent care clinic.
- Have the patient visit the post-acute care clinic.
- Send a home health nurse or therapist to the patient's home.
- Have the patient or caregiver contact a pharmacist to answer medication questions.
- Contact a family member to discuss ways to provide additional support and alternative care options.
- Transfer the patient directly to the SNF, long-term acute care hospital, or acute rehabilitation hospital if the patient was discharged from the hospital in the prior 30 days.

If the situation is not an emergency, the goal is to contact someone who can provide necessary information, help, or comfort while avoiding an unnecessary hospital readmission. Home care agencies and private-duty nurses should be advocates for the idea that home-based care and services play an important role in preventing unnecessary hospital readmissions.

REFER ALL PATIENTS TO HOME CARE OR PRIVATE-DUTY NURSING ON DISCHARGE FROM HOME HEALTH

The discharge from home health services to home care or a private-duty nurse represents the handoff between post-acute care and a healthy lifestyle or wellness. Discharging a patient from home health services indicates that the patient has reached full recovery, has plateaued and can no longer benefit from these services, or is no longer covered by an insurance or Medicare benefit for home health services. Although a patient might continue to receive therapy on an outpatient basis or visit a physician's office for a specific need, once the home health episode concludes, all home-based care must to be paid for by the patient because the insurer is no longer responsible for these services. Because the patient pays for such services, a physician's order is not required. Of course, the patient can and often does refuse home care or private-duty nursing services, but it is still in the best interests of the patient, hospital, and payer for all patients to be referred for home-based support.

IMPLEMENT TRANSFERS DIRECTLY FROM THE ED TO HOME WITH HOME CARE OR PRIVATE-DUTY NURSE SUPPORT

Most healthcare leaders assume that patients are discharged from the ED to home with an order for support services in the home. However, this practice was rare in the fee-for-service model, where physicians and hospitals were incentivized to admit patients. In contrast, in the post-ACA model, this practice will be common. The safest way to discharge patients home and eliminate concern and liability is to do so with a home health order and with coordinated home care support.

EQUIP FAMILY MEMBERS AND FRIENDS TO SERVE AS CARETAKERS

Dr. Eric Coleman (2014), designer of Care Transitions Interventions, asserts that his next focus in the readmissions issue will be caretakers. He says we need to better equip caretakers to help solve the readmission problem. Many of the tactics discussed in this book can also be used to educate family members as caretakers, including teach-back, patient health literacy, and basic medication management knowledge.

My mother was diagnosed with Alzheimer's disease in 2010, and my family's story may shed some light on how families can be involved in caretaking and preventing readmissions. After 45 years of marriage, my father was faced with the challenge of caring for his lifelong partner as her memory eroded and her confusion increased. At a recent family meeting, we discussed how best to care for my mother and ensure her safety when my father was at work. Each family member had a different perspective on this topic. Though it seemed to be time to hire a home care agency or private-duty nurse, my father was hesitant. He preferred to have his children and their spouses take turns providing support. Although we were all willing to commit to this plan of care, I was adamant that if we were not going to hire professional caretakers, then we at least needed to consult with professionals to obtain useful tools, protocols, and resources. Thus, I encouraged my father to hire a home care agency or private-duty nurse initially so that we could learn from their professional experience and expertise.

In addition to Dr. Coleman's research findings on caretakers (www.caretransitions.org), readers may want to look at Care at Hand (www.careathand.com), a tool that CEO Andre Ostrovsky explains was developed to provide caretakers with additional support in the home.

SUMMARY

Although only the most progressive of health systems are currently investing in home care and private-duty caretaking options, health systems as a whole will soon start to implement a model in which discharge to home is the first option. This model will be a result of the incentives, penalties, and programs in the ACA. Thus, a significant opportunity lies ahead for home health agencies and home care agencies, and the operational and marketing tactics identified in this chapter and its accompanying Perspectives will position a home care or private-duty nursing agency to rise above its competition and become the provider of choice. It will then be a key partner in reducing unnecessary hospital readmissions and a preferred provider of home-based services that will thrive in the post-ACA model.

PERSPECTIVE
Preventing Readmissions Through Home Visits

By Jay Licuanan, MD
Vice president and medical director, PA House Calls

Over the past few decades, house calls have been considered an old-fashioned approach to caring for patients. Most private practices were office based as a result of such factors as increasing patient volume and the emergence of the computer age. Early technological advances were not portable and, as a result, rooted physicians in the office. This model of outpatient care persisted until recently.

The advent of healthcare reform was spurred by multiple factors, including inaccessibility to care, increasing administrative costs, and extravagant healthcare spending. Reform has scrutinized every aspect of the troubled

→

---

healthcare system and introduced initiatives to address its problems. One emerging trend in the healthcare reform movement has been an increase in the number of physicians who have returned to performing house calls for such reasons as improved quality of care and diversification of the practice.

Medical groups specializing in this form of healthcare delivery have sprouted up in many states. Collaboratives have been formed among hospitals, home health providers, and house call providers to reduce readmissions through transitional care programs. Home visits have been shown to improve outcomes through continuity of care and increased patient satisfaction, and they have also demonstrated the potential to reduce healthcare costs through the use of various types of providers, including physicians, physician assistants, and nurse practitioners.

Health plans have now recognized the benefits of a transitional care program that incorporates house calls. Major insurance companies, such as Aetna and Cigna, have begun to coordinate and contract for house calls to manage patients who are at high risk for readmission.

As we move forward with the intricacies of reform, it has become apparent that house calls can meet many challenges, particularly those related to the issue of 30-day hospital readmissions. The house-call model is designed to address the key factors in successfully preventing hospital readmissions. The provider is able to visit the patient within the crucial 72-hour period after discharge. Medication reconciliation can be reviewed with the patient and family or caretaker. Education is initiated at the first visit and continued through subsequent visits. Finally, establishing an open line of communication over the first three days can help to identify and resolve medical issues.

→

This full spectrum of the patient–physician interaction occurs in the privacy and comfort of the patient's home. The more relaxed environment eliminates the pressures, time constraints, and sterility commonly associated with an office visit. It creates an atmosphere more conducive to learning and improved understanding of such areas as medication management and chronic medical conditions, and it fosters a better relationship between the patient and the provider.

Clearly, the age-old house call has once again taken an important position in the healthcare landscape. The difference now lies in its complexity in delivering care and in its objective to provide high-quality, cost-conscious care that ultimately reduces hospital readmissions.

PERSPECTIVE
Reducing Psychiatric Readmissions from the Emergency Department

By Leslie S. Zun, MD
System chair, Department of Emergency Medicine,
Sinai Health System, Chicago

Certain risk factors place psychiatric patients at risk for readmission, including low-level schooling, younger age, schizophrenia, personality disorder, use of psychoactive substances, male gender, number of prior hospitalizations, living conditions, number of times the patient is admitted per year, eligibility for disability benefits, and the lack of a discharge plan from a primary care provider. The readmission problem is particularly acute in the elderly population. Elderly patients who have prior hospitalizations for substance use,

→

psychiatric comorbidities, poisoning, adverse drug reactions, and falls are at high risk for being readmitted.

Another category of psychiatric patients who are often readmitted to the hospital are those with suicidal ideation. Suicide ideation and attempts are commonly associated with substance use disorder, personality disorder, prior psychiatric admission, unemployment, and receipt of social benefits. The last group of frequently readmitted psychiatric patients includes patients with lower patient satisfaction, those living with others, and those with poor global functioning. The readmission problem is also found with pediatric patients who have a psychiatric illness. These patients are usually readmitted within 90 days of the initial diagnosis. Factors for readmission include conduct problems, harsh parental discipline, disengaged parents, and parents' stress level.

A number of measures can be taken to reduce readmission for psychiatric patients who come through the emergency department (ED). One tactic is to analyze patients who are chronic users of the ED and who are frequently readmitted to the hospital. This analysis can be done by examining admission diagnoses, presenting complaints, and comments of admitting and ED physicians. For these patients, an action plan to reduce ED use and readmissions is essential. The first step is to determine why the patient returns to the ED. The analysis commonly shows a communication error, inability to obtain follow-up resources, and unmet social needs. The solution is to embed a social worker and mental health worker into the ED to determine the best means of care.

Many patients present to the ED because they have nowhere else to go to resolve their dispute or social situation. Nursing

→

homes, the police (for persons in custody), group homes, and even families may send a patient to the ED not because she is in psychiatric crisis but because she was involved in an altercation or a disagreement that could not be resolved. These institutions are concerned about liability in keeping such patients in their care setting. Other times patients are brought to the ED because no other appropriate community resources are available to resolve their issues. These issues may include lack of housing, need for medication, or the need to find an appropriate care provider. When these patients come to the ED, the staff there may have difficulty contacting the provider, psychiatrists, or others to obtain collateral information needed to send the patient back to his current care setting.

The decision to admit psychiatric patients who come to the ED is not an easy one. No set criteria are available to determine if the patient needs to be admitted. The hard criteria are risk to self, risk to others, or inability to care for oneself. Often, patients do not fit into these categories, making the treatment decision more difficult. Various scoring systems can be used to determine if a patient needs to be admitted. One system uses decision support with three criteria: suicide potential, danger to others, and severity of symptoms. This decision-support system has been found to predict 75 percent of admissions (Lyons et al. 1997). Another tool, the crisis triage rating scale, assesses three criteria (dangerousness, support system, ability to cooperate) on a scale of one to five. A patient with a total score of eight or less needs to be admitted.

The use of mobile crisis units, telepsychiatry, and proper suicide risk assessment are other means to determine if a patient needs to be admitted. Telepsychiatry, which is useful in communities that have limited or no psychiatric resources,

→

can be used for a variety of diagnoses, ages, and complaints and can provide consultation, assessment, medication management, and even family and patient psychotherapy in the ED.

Many ED physicians believe that all patients who at some point in their life have mentioned suicide ideation need to be admitted. For some of those patients, however, an admission may be detrimental. Rather, an appropriate risk assessment for suicidal tendencies needs to be obtained. Although no risk assessment tool is perfect, there are means to properly identify those at high risk who need admission, those at moderate risk who need psychiatric consultation, and those at low risk who may go home.

If it is determined that a patient needs to be admitted, alternatives to inpatient admission may be considered. Brief admission programs, day hospitals, crisis respite, and observational care and crisis stabilization units provide alternatives to admission. The most successful of these programs is the crisis stabilization unit, where patients are assessed, medicated, and referred to community resources within 24 hours of presentation. These units have been reported to reduce admissions and readmissions by 70 percent.

Alternatively, patients may receive treatment or other services in the ED, including rapid response, brief interventions, enhanced interventions, and crisis planning. These interventions have primarily focused on suicidal adolescents who can benefit by brief intervention and enhanced follow-up.

Patients who are sent home need a clear discharge plan that is detailed; is tailored to the patient, family, and clinicians; and contains a safety plan. Telehealth may be used to provide

→

home monitoring. The ED physician, nurse, social worker, or pharmacist may follow up with the patient by phone shortly after discharge. A patient navigator may also help ensure that the patient gets proper support and guidance throughout the healthcare continuum. Studies have shown that use of navigators to guide patients through the healthcare system reduces readmissions (Balaban et al. 2013).

One of the best ways to ensure a patient is not readmitted is to make sure he receives the proper intervention while hospitalized. Other approaches that have significantly reduced readmissions include pre- and postdischarge patient education, structured needs assessment, medication reconciliation, use of transition managers, inpatient and outpatient communication, outpatient follow-up, and attendance at activities. For patients who are noncompliant in taking their oral daily medications, long-acting intramuscular medications should be considered.

In summary, psychiatric patients commonly come to the ED and are admitted (or readmitted) to the hospital. Providers need to properly assess, treat, and connect the patient with outpatient and community psychiatric resources to reduce these readmissions. The ED can play a key role in reducing readmissions for many patients, but particularly for psychiatric patients.

REFERENCES

Balaban, R., A. Galbraith, M. Burns, C. Vialle-Valentin, E. Friedman, and D. Ross-Degnan. 2013. "A Randomized Controlled Trial of a Patient Navigator Intervention to Reduce Hospital Readmissions in a Safety Net Health Care System." *Clinical Medicine & Research* 11 (3): 157–58.

Coleman, E. 2014. Conversation with the author, June 3.

Lyons, J. S., J. Stutesman, J. Neme, J. T. Vessey, M. T. O'Mahoney, and H. J. Camper. 1997. "Predicting Psychiatric Emergency Admissions and Hospital Outcome." *Medical Care* 35 (8): 792–800.

Part V

EPILOGUE

Readmission Prevention Tactics Are Just the First Step in Transforming to a Patient-Focused Delivery System

As stated in Chapter 1, the objective of this book is to provide tactics, tools, and resources that will help healthcare operators prevent unnecessary hospital readmissions. Even if you find only one tactic in this book that applies to your affiliated organization, put it to work! Discuss the tactic with your staff, strategize on how to implement it, and operationalize it. Regardless of the level of care, all healthcare operators are faced with this new challenge of preventing unnecessary readmissions.

Although many health networks will implement many of these tactics, not all hospitals have an abundance of resources readily available to address multiple new initiatives and to create multiple new programs. Many hospitals struggle to survive from one day to the next. I wrote this book to provide hope for administrators who have accepted the challenge of leading facilities and pioneering readmission prevention efforts. Those who are willing to lead the charge to transform their organization to a patient-centered delivery model must be creative in identifying and using resources to achieve their goals in a cost-effective way.

Whether you lead a health system with a mature care coordination plan that uses several of the tactics discussed in this book, a safety-net hospital that has yet to implement a readmission prevention plan, or a post-acute care provider that is seeking to find the best way to support its local hospital in preventing readmissions, this book has something for you. My hope is that you found the discussion of the tactics to be educational and beneficial whether or not you choose to implement any of them.

I am often asked if the Centers for Medicare & Medicaid Services (CMS) will increase the readmission penalty beyond 3 percent in fiscal year 2016. My answer is always the same: Whether or not CMS increases the percentage of the penalty or expands the number of diseases included in the penalty is not the point. What is important to understand is that CMS will continue to find ways to penalize hospitals that admit patients who could have been cared for at a lower level of care. Understanding the concept behind readmission penalties is the key to understanding the overall mind-set of CMS.

When I started writing this book, the Affordable Care Act had five initiatives that incentivize or penalize hospitals for effectively coordinating care. With the launch of the Medicare Spending per Beneficiary measurement and penalty in October 2014, there are now six programs with financial implications for providers that do not effectively coordinate care and avoid admitting patients who could be cared for at a lower level of care. In addition, readmission penalties for skilled-nursing facilities will be introduced in the coming years. Each of these programs has financial implications that point back to the goal of keeping people out of institutions if they can be cared for at home.

Whether or not these programs are expanded or new programs are created that emphasize coordinated care, CMS is going to great lengths to end the practices and protocols that evolved as a result of the fee-for-service reimbursement model. In a world where hospitals will only be paid for patients who could not have been cared for at a lower level of care, emergency department protocols are being turned upside down as physicians are taught to ask first if they can get the patient home and not if they can justify admitting the patient to the hospital. The sooner your hospital can create a "how soon can we get this patient home?" mind-set in its outpatient settings, in the emergency department, and on inpatient units, the sooner your hospital culture will align with the financial incentives of the Affordable Care Act.

In the Appendixes you will find tools and case examples that will be beneficial in your efforts to reduce readmission. For additional best-practice case studies in readmission prevention, visit the National Readmission Prevention Collaborative website (www.nationalreadmissionprevention.com). Readmission prevention tool kits and resources are available on the website, and you can submit your facility's readmission prevention success story for posting as a best-practice case study. Other websites with resources and tools include INTERACT (Interventions to Reduce Acute Care Transfers) (http://interact2.net), COMS Interactive (www.ComsInteractive.com), Care Patrol (www.CarePatrol.com), Medline (www.Medline.com), Care Centrix (http://carecentrix .com), and Health Services Advisory Group (www.hsag.com).

Appendix A

READMISSION TOOLS FOR ACUTE AND POST-ACUTE CARE PROVIDERS

Tool 1. Hospital Skilled-Nursing Facility Discharge Tracking Log

Dec-14	Total	Medicare	Medicaid	Managed Care	No Pay/ Cash	Private Pay	Hospice	Others
Hospital TCU	123	48	0	20	28	26	1	0
SNF 1	2	0	0	1	0	0	0	1
SNF 2	10	7	1	1	0	0	1	0
SNF 3	4	4	0	0	0	0	0	0
SNF 4	20	4	0	2	14	0	0	0
SNF 5	14	14	0	0	0	0	0	0
SNF 6	22	4	2	5	9	2	0	0
SNF 7	18	14	0	4	0	0	0	0
Grand Total	**213**	**95**	**3**	**33**	**51**	**28**	**2**	**1**

Note: TCU = transitional care unit; SNF = skilled-nursing facility.

Use this log to track the volume of post-acute discharges being sent to each facility. This tool can help identify if a doctor or case manager is referring a high volume of patients to one specific facility, as well as if a certain SNF has a high readmission rate and an assessment is needed to determine how significant the hospital's exposure is. An SNF's readmission rate is calculated by dividing the number of readmissions the SNF has to the hospital (the numerator) by the total number of patients admitted to the SNF from the hospital (the denominator).

Tool 2. Readmissions Tracking Log by Post-Acute Care Provider

Dec-14	Total	Dr. A	Dr. B	Dr. C	Dr. D	Case Manager A	Case Manager B	Case Manager C
Hospital TCU	123	48	0	20	28	26	0	0
SNF 1	2	0	0	1	0	0	0	1
SNF 2	10	7	1	1	0	0	1	0
LTAC Hospital 1	4	4	0	0	0	0	0	0
LTAC Hospital 2	20	4	0	2	14	0	0	0
Home Health A	14	14	0	0	0	0	0	0
Home Health B	22	4	2	5	9	2	0	0
IRF 1	18	14	0	4	0	0	0	0
IRF 2	14	14	0	0	0	0	0	0
Hospice A	22	4	2	5	9	2	0	0
Hospice B	18	14	0	4	0	0	0	0
ALF 1	14	14	0	0	0	0	0	0
ALF 2	14	14	0	0	0	0	0	0
Grand Total	**295**	**155**	**5**	**42**	**60**	**30**	**1**	**1**

Notes: TCU = transitional care unit; SNF = skilled-nursing facility; LTAC = long-term acute care; IRF = inpatient rehabilitation facility; ALF = assisted-living facility.

Ask your hospital partners to implement this tracking log so they can better manage their own physician and case manager referral patterns. It may be a tough sell, but their systems can generate a similar report if you ask. They may not be willing to share this information with you, but don't let that stop you from suggesting they track it!

Tool 3. Monthly Readmissions Dashboard

Month: December (data ending 12/31/14)	Acute Discharges	Readmission Percentage	YTD	Prior Year	Current Quarter to Date	1Q	2Q	3Q	4Q	Current Month	Prior Month
Medicare FFS											
MCR FFS All Diagnoses	377	9.28%									
MCR FFS AMI		0.00%									
MCR FFS CHF		0.00%									
MCR FFS COPD		0.00%									
MCR FFS Pneumonia		0.00%									
MCR FFS Total Knee/Hip		0.00%									
MCR FFS Nonpenalty Diagnosis											
Other MCR FFS	377	9.28%									

(continued)

Tool 3. Monthly Readmissions Dashboard (continued)

Managed Medicare Product A									
Managed Medicare Product B									
MCR FFS—DC Disposition									
Discharge to Home/Self-Care	148	10.14%							
Discharge/Transfer to Outside SNF	66	7.58%							
Discharge/Transfer to Other Acute Care Hospital	2								
Discharge/Transfer to SNF DP	57	15.79%							
Discharge/Transfer to Home Health	103	5.83%							
Discharge/Transfer to Outside Psych	1								

(continued)

Discharge/Transfer to Board and Care	7						
Discharge/Transfer to Hospice Home	7						
Left Against Medical Advice	2						
Discharge/Transfer to Other Acute Floor	7						
Death	16						
Discharge/Transfer to Outside Rehab	7						
Discharge/Transfer to Outside LTAC Hospital	2						

Notes: YTD = year to date; MCR = Medicare; FFS = fee for service; AMI = acute myocardial infarction; CHF = congestive heart failure; COPD = chronic obstructive pulmonary disease; DC = discharge; SNF = skilled-nursing facility; DP = distinct part; LTAC = long-term acute care.

This dashboard provides a real-time analysis of a hospital's readmissions by showing baseline and historical data for comparison. A hospital's readmission rate is calculated by dividing the number of readmissions to the hospital (the numerator) by the total number of patients discharged from the hospital (the denominator).

Tool 4. Skilled-Nursing Facility Intake Log

SNF or Agency Name

Hospital Name

Month/Year: _____ Week Ending: _____

Resident Name	Payer	Admit Date	Admitting Physician	Discharging Case Manager	Discharge Date	Discharge Disposition

Notes: SNF = skilled-nursing facility.

SNFs can use this tool to log individual admissions from each hospital and thus track how many of those patients end up being readmitted to the hospital.

Tool 5. Return to Emergency Department Log

SNF or Agency Name					Month/Year:			Week Ending:
Resident Name	Payer	Admit Date	Return to Hospital Date	Reason	Charge Nurse at Time of Readmission	Disposition	INTERACT Care Paths Followed	Root-Cause Analysis Performance Improvement Findings

Note: SNF = skilled-nursing facility.

Use this form to document all patients who return to any hospital for any reason, even if they are not readmitted. Any patient who leaves the facility should be logged.

Appendix B

CASE EXAMPLES

Einstein Medical Center: Medication REACH Program

By Mariel Sjeime, PharmD
Transition of care pharmacist,
Einstein Healthcare Network, Philadelphia

CHALLENGE ADDRESSED

Einstein Medical Center in Philadelphia, Pennsylvania, serves a large, vulnerable safety-net population and is at risk of declining reimbursement if key performance-oriented metrics for hospital readmissions are not met. The costs associated with the current healthcare delivery system are unsustainable, which has led to new emerging models.

NEEDS ASSESSMENT

Medication-related errors are common during transitions between healthcare settings. About 50 percent of all hospital-related medication errors and 20 percent of adverse drug events are attributed to poor communication during transitions of care (American Pharmacists Association and American Society of Health-System Pharmacists 2012), and 30 to 70 percent of medication discrepancies occur at hospital admission (Jack et al. 2009). Low health literacy complicates the problem further. Medication nonadherence has been referred to as the Achilles' heel of modern healthcare (Vermeire et al. 2002), and studies have shown that 20 to 50 percent of patients do not take prescription medications as directed (Kripalani et al. 2007). Medication nonadherence accounts for 10 percent of all hospital admissions (Hubbard and McNeill 2012) at an annual estimated cost between $100 and $300 billion (Walker 2001).

PROCESS CREATED

Einstein Medical Center conducted a prospective controlled study funded by the Albert Einstein Society and approved by the institutional review board. The goal was to enhance the patient discharge process through multidisciplinary communication and direct pharmacist involvement in an effort to reduce adverse medication events and hospital readmissions. We developed a process called Medication REACH, where the *R* stands for *reconciliation*—that is, the pharmacist validates the medication reconciliation to ensure completeness and accuracy. The *E* stands for the *education* the pharmacist provides patients about their medications. The *A* represents the myriad issues surrounding *access* to care. The *C* refers to the follow-up *counseling* patients receive after discharge. Finally, the *H* symbolizes a *healthy patient at home*, which is our ultimate goal.

Pharmacy residents at Einstein Medical Center partnered with the care management department to identify patients who met the following criteria: 18 years old or older, taking five or more medications, more than one chronic condition, 48 hours or more of hospitalization, discharges to home, and admission to telemetry or cardiac care unit. These patients formed the study group that would participate in the Medication REACH program. Pharmacy residents then validated the medication reconciliation at admission and at discharge to optimize the medication regimen. Patients were provided with patient-centered education, a medication list, and a pillbox. Pharmacy residents ensured that prescriptions were filled at our discharge pharmacy or the patient's local pharmacy and made a follow-up phone call once within 72 hours of discharge; after that, the pharmacist called the patient weekly over the 30 days after discharge. The control group was discharged according to the facility's usual procedures.

OUTCOMES ACHIEVED

The readmission rates for patients participating in Medication REACH were nearly half of those for the control group (see Exhibit A.1). Pharmacists performed 59 interventions in the 47 patients in the study group (see Exhibit A.2). The large number and variety of interventions indicate that there is tremendous opportunity for pharmacists to improve the medication regimen.

Exhibit A.1 30-Day Readmission Rates

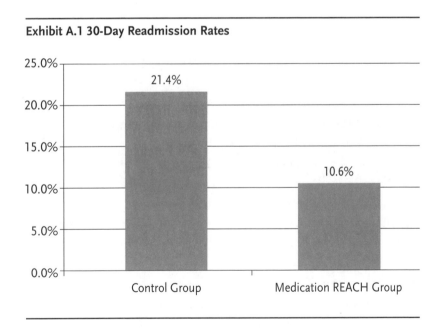

Exhibit A.2 Pharmacist Interventions

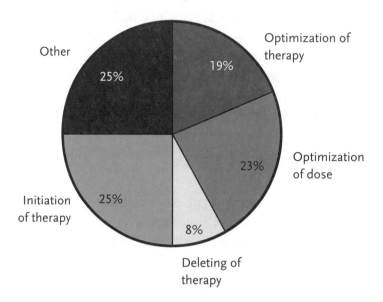

Total number of patients = 47   Total number of interventions = 59

EXPANSIONS AND ENHANCEMENTS

Since the Medication REACH program began in 2010, we have opened a discharge pharmacy to service all discharged patients. We have also hired a full-time transition-of-care pharmacist. To allow the pharmacist to reach as many patients as possible and focus on clinical responsibilities, we developed two advanced pharmacy technician roles. The first role, called *ambulatory pharmacy patient liaison empowerment,* or APPLE, helps resolve access-to-care issues at discharge. Next, we created a medication reconciliation technician role in the emergency department with the goal of decreasing medication errors on admission. We have also partnered with other organizations and delegated responsibilities to other healthcare professionals to reach as many patients as possible.

ACKNOWLEDGMENTS

Special thanks to Angelo DeLuca, PharmD, associate director of clinical services; Leonard Braitman, PhD, biostatistician; Priscilla Mooney, PharmD, manager of Einstein Apothecary; and Einstein Medical Center's pharmacy residents for all of their hard work in implementing Medication REACH.

REFERENCES

American Pharmacists Association and American Society of Health-System Pharmacists. 2012. "Improving Care Transitions: Optimizing Medication Reconciliation." Published March. www.pharmacist.com/sites/default/files/files/2012_improving_care_transitions.pdf.

Hubbard, T., and N. McNeill. 2012. "Improving Medication Adherence and Reducing Readmissions." Network for Excellence in Health Innovation issue brief. Published October. www.nacds.org/pdfs/pr/2012/nehi-readmissions.pdf.

Jack, B. W., V. K. Chetty, D. Anthony, J. L. Greenwald, G. M. Sanchez, A. E. Johnson, S. R. Forsythe, J. K. O'Donnell, M. K. Paasche-Orlow, C. Manasseh, S. Martin, and L. Culpepper. 2009. "A Reengineered Hospital Discharge Program to Decrease Rehospitalization." *Annals of Internal Medicine* 150 (3): 178–87.

Kripalani, S., S. Robertson, M. H. Love-Ghaffari, L. E. Henderson, J. Praska, A. Strawder, M. G. Katz, and T. A. Jacobson. 2007. "Development of an Illustrated Medication Schedule as a Low-Literacy Patient Education Tool." *Patient Education and Counseling* 66 (3): 368–77.

Vermeire, E., H. Hearnshaw, P. Van Royen, and J. Denekens. 2002. "Patient Adherence to Treatment: Three Decades of Research. A Comprehensive Review." *Journal of Clinical Pharmacy and Therapeutics* 26 (5): 331–42.

Walker, T. 2001. "Understanding Patients' Needs Is Key to Medication Compliance." *Managed Healthcare Executive* 11 (1): 34.

Lee Memorial Health System: Comprehensive Care Transitions Program

By Christine Nesheim
System director, care management,
Lee Memorial Health System, Fort Myers, Florida

Over the past three years, Lee Memorial Health System (LMHS) in Fort Myers, Florida, has built a comprehensive program for care transitions to improve quality and reduce costs. The program's success is measured at the highest level by the 30-day all-cause readmission rates. Data from LMHS's participation in the Florida Hospital Association / Florida Medical Quality Assurance Inc. collaborative, No Place Like Home, demonstrate that Lee Memorial Hospital and HealthPark Medical Center, two of the acute care hospitals in LMHS, have reached a 15.9 percent readmission rate, which is better than the national (18.2 percent) and Florida (18.9 percent) readmission rates. Specific readmission reductions for acute myocardial infarction and congestive heart failure (CHF) exceeded the first-year goal after only six months in the collaborative.

To help achieve readmission reduction goals, LMHS tracks and analyzes readmission and discharge data and learns from national best practices. The organization has also revamped services from admission through acute care treatment and has improved efforts to educate and empower patients. The program combines high-tech and high-touch components, and we have already transferred successful program components to other hospitals, skilled-nursing facilities (SNFs), assisted-living facilities, home health agencies, and patient homes. We developed an original high-risk stratification tool to be used at admission to quickly assess patient risks and set standards for specific care while a patient is hospitalized and when they are discharged. Finally, teach-back education was provided to nursing and case managers system-wide and to several home health agencies.

HealthPark Medical Center has been accredited as a CHF center and is opening an observation unit for diaphoresis and discharge. At discharge, several care pathways are available: telehealth remote monitoring, a care transitions personal coach, or Interventions to Reduce Acute Care Transfers (INTERACT) II–supported care at SNFs.

Telehealth remote patient monitoring through Lee Memorial Home Health combines technology with high-quality medical attention to provide home medical management. Currently, more than 250 patients use remote patient monitors, and more than 6,000 patients have been monitored since the program launched in 2010. Data show that the 30-day readmission rate for all telehealth patients is 9 percent. The success was featured as a best practice by our national technology partner, Honeywell.

LMHS also trained care transition nurse coaches to meet with patients before discharge and then at home with their caregiver to address medical concerns, medication discrepancies, red flags for the patient's condition, safety issues, and setting-specific personal health goals. Home medication discrepancies dropped from 80 percent to 5 percent when the program was pilot-tested at HealthPark Medical Center. A binder labeled "My Personal Health Record" is provided for documentation and for patient education in the hospital and at home. The 30-day readmission rate for patients assigned to a care transitions personal coach is now 11 percent.

Educational handouts for CHF, chronic obstructive pulmonary disease (COPD), and pneumonia have been standardized and are used system-wide. A COPD program is in its third month of trial, and of 19 patients (who had repetitive readmissions), only one was readmitted.

LMHS partnered with SNFs and home health agencies to develop a community collaborative and action plan. On discharge, patients return or transition to an SNF, assisted-living facility, or hospice facility. To improve quality care and reduce readmissions, LMHS adopted the quality improvement program INTERACT II. LMHS staff who are INTERACT certified are training community facilities to use the INTERACT tools to focus on acute changes in resident conditions. Seventeen area SNFs have completed the training and meet monthly to discuss process implementation, barriers, and education. Since the implementation of INTERACT II, skilled-nursing readmissions decreased from 20 percent to 17.5 percent. INTERACT III training was rolled out to area assisted-living facilities and home health companies in 2014.

A Stanford University best-practice program for chronic disease self-management was implemented in a train-the-trainer approach with social service agencies, which would then provide six weeks of education to residents of the care facility with the goal of improving the overall health of patients with chronic conditions. The program has resulted in a 20 percent decrease in costly emergency department visits and a 10 percent decrease in hospital readmissions.

We have also implemented two programs that focus on preventing malnutrition in high-risk and indigent patients after discharge—the Fresh at Home meal delivery pilot and a partnership with the Harry Chapin Food Bank to provide patients with vouchers to area food banks. Furthermore, the Lee Physician Group, which includes more than 300 primary and specialty care physicians, is implementing the medical home model and should be certified soon.

With enthusiastic staff and with patient and community support, we continue to expand the depth and breadth of LMHS's system-wide Comprehensive Care Transitions Program.

Los Alamitos Medical Center: Preventing Readmissions Collaborative

By Debbie Rivet
Case management director, Los Alamitos Medical Center,
Los Alamitos, California

The Preventing Readmissions Group, a working coalition of health-care professionals in Los Alamitos, California, meets monthly at Los Alamitos Medical Center to discuss the concerns and needs of the community and hospital. The group's motivating focus is to improve patient care and reduce readmissions. During the meetings, members share how readmissions affect their particular agency and the overall effect those readmissions have on the hospital. The result since the inception of the readmissions group is a reduction in preventable readmissions of approximately 10 percent.

The first meeting in the fall of 2011 was attended by about 15 people, including the administrators of two local community skilled-nursing facilities (SNFs) and a local home health agency, as well as the hospital's director of case management; chief nursing officer; coronary artery disease coordinator; director of quality support services; nursing directors from the intensive care unit, emergency department, and medical surgical units; social workers; dietary clinicians; and the director of pharmacy. The group, which had grown to about 45 people as of June 2014, is now open to anyone in the local healthcare community.

The group's initial goals were to evaluate and analyze readmission scores and to create and implement a community-based support system that is united in using an evidence-based approach to reducing hospital readmissions. Decreasing readmission rates for acute myocardial infarction, congestive heart failure, and pneumonia were among the first goals of the group, and other goals have included improving transitions of care, sharing concerns about level of care and processes, implementing evidence-based approaches such as Project RED (Re-Engineered Discharge), and educating healthcare workers in all settings—from hospitals to SNFs, long-term acute care hospitals, home health, hospice, and durable medical equipment—as well as other stakeholders in this transition-of-care community approach.

The Preventing Readmissions Group complements the mission of the Tenet Readmission Advisory Committee (TRAC) by also being patient centered; focusing on the best care, the right place, and the right team; and establishing collaborations. The Preventing Readmissions Group educates the community about how to help prevent avoidable readmissions and brings updates to TRAC as warranted. Every month the group does a root-cause analysis to identify at least one vulnerability in the delivery system and how it directly affects patient care and potential risks for admission.

New programs have come about as a result of the Preventing Readmissions Group. For example, the respiratory department developed an education program for SNFs. Classes are also available for SNFs and other post-acute care providers to learn about congestive heart failure and coronary artery disease, concentrating on the topics of tests, medications, nutrition, exercise and activity, and coping. The group also developed a comprehensive brochure explaining the clinical capabilities available at the different levels of care; this brochure was introduced to the community and physician's offices to serve as a resource for patients and providers.

The Preventing Readmissions Collaborative has successfully improved patient care and reduced readmissions through a collaborative effort of various members of the community. These goals were accomplished by syncing the collaborative's efforts with the missions of other groups, such as TRAC.

Omnicare: A Program to Reduce Rehospitalizations and Improve Quality of Care in Medicare Beneficiaries on Admission to the Nursing Home

By Barbara J. Zarowitz, PharmD
Chief clinical officer and vice president of clinical services,
Omnicare Inc.

BACKGROUND

Medication reconciliation and elimination of potentially unnecessary medications reduce avoidable adverse drug events. The pilot program examined how these interventions at the time of nursing home admission affected quality and rehospitalization rates in a 100-bed skilled-nursing facility (SNF) of Medicare beneficiaries in Cincinnati, Ohio.

METHODS

The program was implemented using a prospective, concurrent study design. As part of the program, the SNF nurse liaison faxed hospital discharge information to a clinical pharmacist for review, medication reconciliation, and recommended intervention as soon as notification of a potential admission was received. After medication reconciliation and before admission to the SNF, pharmacists prepared a set of admission medication orders that eliminated duplicate medications, set stop dates where appropriate, adjusted doses to prevent renal impairment, offered lower-cost alternatives that were comparatively safe and effective, and corrected drug omissions. These orders were reviewed and authorized by the SNF physician. Data for each admission were collected, and cost avoidance was calculated per 30 days using facility acquisition cost and nursing time avoided.

RESULTS

In 38 sequential admissions over two months, 241 interventions resulted in an 87 percent reduction in use of high-risk medications, 97 drug discontinuations or dosage reductions, 45 drug changes, 16 reductions in duration of therapy, and one readmission (for a readmission rate of 2.6 percent). Frequent interventions included elimination of sliding-scale insulin, proton pump inhibitors, and antipsychotic medications. Clinical quality improvements resulted from a reduction in redundant antidiabetic medications and high-risk, high-cost anti-coagulant therapy. These interventions resulted in an average savings of $249 per admission in unnecessary drug costs and nursing time (30 minutes per admission) associated with medication reconciliation and transcription. Nurses reported high satisfaction with the service because they were more available to perform patient assessment and provide care. Medication availability was expedited and monitored by the clinical pharmacy team (an average of 1.7 hours per admission) from the point of data acquisition, medication reconciliation, order verification, and authorization to the point of order entry in the pharmacy and medication fulfillment and delivery.

CONCLUSIONS

By prospectively conducting medication reconciliation and performing medication therapy management before admission, we identified and avoided many potentially unnecessary medications and excessive durations of therapy after hospital discharge. Key features of the program were the strength of the partnership between the medical staff, nursing staff, and pharmacists. Because medication-related events were preemptively aborted, the improvement in quality and efficiency was heralded by the facility staff as an improvement in medication safety, too. Streamlining therapy may have contributed to reduced rehospitalizations and fewer falls during the months of the pilot program.

UCLA Health System:
A Collaborative Approach
to Reducing Readmissions

By Sarah Lonowski, senior project manager and
quality specialist, UCLA Health System;
and Nasim Afsar-manesh, MD, associate chief medical officer,
UCLA Hospitals, Los Angeles

Reprinted with permission from *Readmission News.*

READMISSIONS: A COMPLEX PROBLEM

Reducing 30-day hospital readmissions has been identified as an important strategy in improving overall quality of care, increasing patient satisfaction, and reducing healthcare costs. Growing public awareness about the negative impact of readmissions and new Centers for Medicare & Medicaid Services (CMS) penalties for hospitals with excess readmissions have prompted hospitals and health systems to take a closer look at their readmission rates.

Yet, as more literature on the subject emerges, it is becoming increasingly clear that reducing hospital readmissions is not a simple task because a readmission can result from any combination of factors occurring throughout the continuum of care, both inpatient and outpatient. For the UCLA Health System, reducing readmissions presents an additional challenge because of the complexity of medical conditions in the patient population. Thus, preventing readmissions means involving and engaging people throughout the continuum of care—the patients in particular, but also their families and caregivers.

THE STRATEGY

UCLA first began to address readmissions in early 2012 with the launch of the health system–wide Readmission Reduction Initiative (RRI). From the outset, the goal of the RRI was to eliminate every single preventable 30-day readmission. To achieve this goal, the health system used a two-part strategy: (1) gain a deep understanding of the readmissions problem in each department, and (2) design and implement targeted interventions based on this understanding.

To gain a thorough understanding of why patients are rehospitalized, departments performed a variety of activities, including patient interviews, root-cause analyses (RCAs), and extensive chart reviews. These types of activities helped shape an accurate and detailed understanding of readmissions at UCLA: Why are patients being readmitted, what resources are needed to provide more comprehensive support, and where are existing gaps in care?

An example helps to illustrate this idea. A patient who presented to the emergency department (ED) was readmitted because she was having uncontrolled pain after surgery. A chart review of the case indicated that the problem was the need for a better pain management plan. Interviewing the patient, however, made it clear that she had attempted to follow up with her outpatient providers for two days but had been unable to reach anyone. As a result, she had come to the ED for pain management. The interview revealed that this particular rehospitalization was in fact a gap in timely outpatient follow-up, not hospital pain management.

Another critical piece of UCLA's strategy was to engage stakeholders across the continuum of care. Such stakeholder engagement was promoted through the formation of a multidisciplinary Readmission Reduction Council, which includes representatives from executive leadership, physicians, nursing, case management, quality, clinical decision support, and others. The council has been instrumental in creating standard health system definitions for readmissions and a comprehensive readmissions dashboard.

Monthly council meetings promote communication and collaboration between departments and across care settings.

THE INTERVENTIONS

Over the first 18 months, the departments engaged in the RRI developed unique, targeted interventions to meet the needs of their patient populations. The following discussion provides a sampling of the interventions implemented across the health system.

The medicine department, for example, created greater awareness of readmissions among providers through the development of accountable care units (ACUs). The ACUs consist of all providers involved in a patient's care during a hospitalization, including physicians, house staff, nurses, and case managers. The ACU is aimed at engaging these providers to conduct a mini-RCA to understand how care could have been improved. The mini-RCA takes the form of a real-time readmission e-mail to the discharging attending physician asking the physician to comment on whether the index hospitalization or the readmission was preventable and, if preventable, what could have been done differently. In the future, the e-mail notification will be sent to all members of the patient's care team.

The orthopedics department achieved decreases in ED utilization and readmission rates through a readmissions, mortality, and sepsis report. Using this report, a multidisciplinary committee meets twice a month to complete a thorough review of all readmissions cases and to identify strategies for preventing future readmissions.

By identifying the most common causes of readmissions, departments have been able to create focused interventions that can significantly reduce readmission rates. The neurosurgery department has curbed ventriculoperitoneal shunt–related readmissions by implementing a preoperative checklist and a supplemental time-out (a hospital tactic used in the operating room to double-check that critical resources are in place and confirm the exact count of each supply) before surgery. Similarly, the general surgery division addressed wound-related readmissions through an in-house postoperative care standardization protocol for colorectal surgery.

Realizing that a significant and sustainable reduction in readmissions requires engagement throughout the continuum of care, UCLA also focused its efforts on the outpatient side through the UCLA Primary Care Innovation Model. As part of primary care redesign, a care coordinator system was implemented in 14 UCLA primary care offices as part of an extensive medical home model. The care coordinator partners with the patient to ensure close follow-up and management of medical and nonclinical issues. Reducing acute care hospital admissions, readmissions, and ED visits is a central goal, and thus far, the program has made significant progress in all areas. The program has been featured in the *New York Times* and *Los Angeles Times* and on *CBS News*.

At a health system level, UCLA is engaged in the Westside Care Transitions Collaborative, a partnership of UCLA, St. John's Hospital, and the Partners in Care Foundation. The collaborative uses CMS funding to implement a nationally recognized coaching model for Medicare patients. The goal is to reduce readmissions by increasing patient knowledge, engagement, and support in the transition from hospital to home.

THE OUTCOME

The work of the RRI is ongoing and has produced interventions that are at various stages of design, development, and implementation. However, preliminary results indicate that these efforts are making an impact. General medicine, general surgery, neurosurgery, pediatrics, and orthopedics have all experienced decreases in their readmission rates since the launch of the RRI (see Exhibit A.3). Overall at UCLA, 30-day readmissions decreased from a 12.2 percent baseline rate to 11.4 percent in the postintervention period.

MOVING FORWARD

As those involved with the RRI continue to work toward the goal of eliminating all preventable readmissions, it is important to recognize and share lessons learned along the way. Members of the Readmission Reduction Council have identified the following key lessons from their work so far:

◆ Understanding the patient population and evaluating current processes are critical in ensuring the implementation of appropriate and effective interventions.

Exhibit A.3 Readmission Rates at UCLA Medical Center Before and After Reduction Initiative, by Department

Department	Baseline (9/2010–12/2011)	Postintervention (1/2012–1/2013)	December 2012
General medicine	20.1%	18.2%	15.6%
General surgery	15.5%	13.4%	13.6%
Neurosurgery	11.0%	10.7%	9.8%
Pediatrics	11.4%	10.9%	10.4%
Orthopaedics	4.4%	4.3%	1.7%

◆ Multidisciplinary teams are essential and must include representatives of all who care for patients in ambulatory and hospital settings, particularly patients and families.
◆ Thinking outside the box helps to develop unique solutions and address readmissions from all possible angles.

With these lessons in mind, UCLA continues working to reduce readmissions and, most important, to provide the best possible care for every patient.

JourneyCare: Palliative Care Reflections on a Readmission Intervention Model

By Kelly Fischer
Chief operating officer, JourneyCare,
Barrington, Illinois

JourneyCare, a small- to mid-sized hospice and palliative care organization in the Chicago area, has a robust palliative care program that is staffed by expert advanced practice nurses (APNs) who serve more than 350 patients and an average hospice census of 500. In June 2012, at a meeting between JourneyCare and a collaborating hospital, the organizations' leaders received challenging feedback. JourneyCare's palliative care program and the hospital's cardiac program were not hitting the target for reducing congestive heart failure (CHF) readmissions.

In response, we at JourneyCare focused attention on the palliative care program and developed an approach to best support the hospital and, most important, the patients and families. With limited resources, we returned to the hospital to collect data and enhance our relationships with the cardiac and discharge teams. Initial meetings were tense. Each organization had limited collaborative problem-solving experience. Establishing transparency among stakeholders was essential. We also needed to troubleshoot the problem and understand the changes in Medicare metrics, which required old systems to produce new data and new patient outcomes. We agreed to develop a trial program to reduce readmissions based on the best available research. We realized that most published studies acknowledged that their outcomes had pros and cons and thus decided to choose the best and translate them into an easy, teach-back engagement for all parties. The result was the program Taking Control of Your Own Health: Palliative Care for Patients with Heart Failure, which was launched in January 2013.

CONTEXT

CHF is the most common cause of hospitalization and rehospitalization for patients older than 65 years. Hospitalization for CHF is common, expensive, and preventable.

OBJECTIVE

The goal in creating the program was to provide an APN post-acute care model to reduce hospital readmissions for this population. Collecting evidence-based data and conducting a meta-analysis of current research and programs were integral to the model's development.

METHODS

We reviewed the available literature from Medline, the Centers for Medicare & Medicaid Services, and the Institute for Healthcare Improvement, as well as all available publications of studies and programs on related topics. Search terms included "congestive heart failure readmission reduction," "current modalities for CHF home management," and "post-acute care—CHF." Publications were selected by three reviewers.

RESULTS

Six studies were selected. In each program, results varied for each of the areas identified as risk factors in reducing readmissions. However, communication problems were identified as an issue across all studies and models. Our analysis resulted in the creation of a patient-empowered, APN consultative hospital/in-home model that would be accompanied by education and communication tools.

The model was constructed in collaboration with a community hospital and had an initial trial period of four months. The true impact was difficult to assess, however, because accurate numbers were not always available for CHF patients admitted for CHF or another reason before the trial. The success rate of the program during the trial period allowed us to extend the trial to one year, and the one-year outcomes continued to show success in reducing hospital readmission rates (see Exhibit A.4).

Exhibit A.4 Number of Hospitalizations Before and After Launch of the CHF Palliative Care Program

	No. (%) of patients	
	Before Pilot (2011–2012)	**After Pilot (Jan. 1, 2013–Jan. 6, 2014)**
Total CHF patients	10	86
Nonhospitalizations	5 (50)	66 (76.7)
Hospitalizations <30 days	1 (10)	13 (15.1)
Hospitalizations 30–60 days	3 (30)	4 (4.7)
Hospitalizations >60 days	11 (110)	3 (3.5)
Total readmissions	15	21
CHF readmissions	1 (6.7)	2 (9.5)
Non-CHF readmissions*	14 (93.3)	19 (90.5)

Note: CHF = congestive heart failure.
*The patient was readmitted for reasons other than a CHF diagnosis.

CONCLUSION

CHF readmissions were notably reduced during the initial four-month period, and reductions in readmissions continued through the full one-year trial, therefore demonstrating the effectiveness of our APN palliative care model in reducing readmissions.

NEXT STEPS

Because of the success of this model, our collaborative partnership is developing an innovative advanced illness model for addressing readmissions for patients with chronic obstructive pulmonary disease.

About the Author

Josh Luke, PhD, FACHE, is founder of the National Readmission Prevention Collaborative and a national thought leader and international speaker on the topics of care coordination, population health management, readmission prevention, and development of integrated post-acute care networks. He is a seasoned hospital CEO, health system vice president, and nursing home administrator. Regarded as a futurist on the Affordable Care Act (ACA) and how it will shape the continuum of care, he has been described as an innovator, a forward thinker, and a strategist on teaching accountable care organizations, bundled-payment initiative programs, and hospital leaders how to position themselves for revenue growth in the transitional care and post-acute care sector in a post-ACA model.

Dr. Luke's broad range of experience with some of the leading companies in healthcare has positioned him as an expert on readmission prevention and care coordination. At the time this book was written, he was serving as the interim CEO of Memorial Hospital of Gardena (California); before that, he served as CEO of Western Medical Center in Anaheim, California, for almost three years and as CEO of Anaheim General Hospital for four years, leading significant financial turnarounds at each facility. After seven years as a hospital CEO, Dr. Luke was named vice president of post-acute care services for Torrance Memorial Health System in Torrance, California. In that role he designed a population management strategy, Total Wellness Torrance, working with accountable care organizations and bundled-payment initiatives. Total Wellness Torrance and its post-acute care network received the Excellence in Programming Award from the California Association of Healthcare Facilities in 2013. Dr. Luke's previous experience also includes serving as CEO of HealthSouth Rehabilitation Hospital of Las Vegas (Nevada) and as an administrator in the skilled-nursing division of Kindred Healthcare in Southern California. He also has experience overseeing assisted-living, home health, and hospice services and is a licensed skilled-nursing facility and Residential Care Facilities for the Elderly administrator and preceptor.

Dr. Luke serves on the executive faculty at California State University–Long Beach in the healthcare administration department. He previously taught at California State University–Fullerton and the University of Phoenix's Nevada campus. Dr. Luke has a doctorate in educational leadership and is a Fellow of the American College of Healthcare Executives. He is a Lean Six Sigma Black Belt and received his Lean certification from Torrance Memorial Health System. He has served as a Lean mentor and project chair and is a past chair of the CalOptima Provider Advisory Committee.

Dr. Luke has served in many advisory and board capacities, including serving on panels with other thought leaders and joining readmission pioneers Dr. Eric Coleman and Dr. Steven Jencks as the third member of a three-person scientific advisory board for a leading organization providing vital services in the home health sector. Other board appointments have included the boards of directors of the California Hospital Association's Center for Post-Acute Care, Hospital Association of Southern California, Healthcare Executives of Southern California, CareCentrix, and Hospice Care of California. He also serves on the California State University–Long Beach Healthcare Administration Advisory Board.

All of this broad experience has made Dr. Luke one of the most sought-after speakers nationally and internationally in teaching health system executives how to create new revenue streams in a post-ACA delivery model. Although many speakers can address anticipated changes as a result of the ACA, Dr. Luke lays out a clear vision of the changes ahead and how best to prepare for them by focusing on the patient. He has served as a consultant for some of the nation's top health systems because he is one of the few people nationally with a successful track record of creating new revenue streams to replace diminishing inpatient census and revenue as the delivery system evolves into a value-based model.

Having founded the National Readmission Prevention Collaborative (www.nationalreadmissionprevention.com) in October 2013 to showcase best-practice integration models, in March 2014 Dr. Luke left his health system job and ventured out on his own as president of the Readmission Prevention Group, working with health systems and communities nationwide to develop post-acute care networks and population health management strategies. In May 2014 Dr. Luke accepted an interim regional administrator position with SNF Management and served in that role for four months; in September 2014 he accepted an interim hospital CEO position with Avanti Hospitals at Memorial Hospital of Gardena in Los Angeles County.

Dr. Luke writes an e-mail newsletter, *NRPC News and Solutions in Population Management, Care Transitions, and Readmissions*, which reaches more than 60,000 healthcare leaders nationwide. He also contributes regularly to the monthly publication *Readmission News* and other healthcare publications. This is Dr. Luke's first book.

About the Contributors

Nasim Afsar-manesh, MD, SFHM, is a practicing hospitalist and chief quality officer in the Department of Medicine at UCLA Health. She has served as the associate chief medical officer at UCLA Health, collaborating with various clinical and nonclinical departments to transform patient care. She has led more than 30 projects in quality, safety, patient satisfaction, efficiency, utilization, and cost, and she has been a pioneer in quality improvement curriculum development, creating a curriculum for the 70 residency and fellowship programs at UCLA accredited by the Accreditation Council for Graduate Medical Education. At the national level, she has been involved in a number of quality and safety efforts, including three multicenter grants from the University of California Office of the President Center for Health Quality and Innovation. She currently serves on the board of directors for the Society of Hospital Medicine and was the past chair of the society's Hospital Quality and Patient Safety Committee.

Hassan Alkhouli, MD, is the chief medical officer for Garden Grove Medical Center in Garden Grove, California, and an internist at Pathway Medical Group in Westminster, California. He completed his residency at Mercy Hospital in Chicago and had a pulmonary fellowship at King Drew Medical Center in Los Angeles. He was a clinical research fellow in the department of anesthesiology at Massachusetts General Hospital in Boston. He is board certified in internal medicine and pulmonary medicine.

Sheetal Amin, PharmD, has been a practicing pharmacist since 1992 and has experience in community and long-term care settings. She is now the owner of Healthy Living Pharmacy in Yorba Linda, California, which opened its doors in 2004. With years of experience as a consultant pharmacist, she is an expert in medication therapy management and works with physicians to prevent readmissions. She also specializes in compounding medications, including but not limited to pain management, bioidentical hormone replacement therapy, and wound and scar care.

Chuck Bongiovanni, MSW, MBA, CSA, CFE, is a nationally recognized speaker on Medicare Spending per Beneficiary (MSPB) measures. He is the author of the Community Integration Model, a model of transitional care that addresses several common reasons for hospital readmissions while simultaneously reducing hospital MSPB measures. The model is rolling out nationally through Medicare Advantage plans, accountable care organizations, hospitals, and hospital systems. Mr. Bongiovanni is also CEO of CarePatrol Franchise Systems, LLC, which helps families find senior housing and is the largest senior assisted-living placement service in the nation. Under his leadership, CarePatrol has been honored by *Inc.* magazine as one of the fastest-growing privately held companies in America, received the coveted Franchisee Satisfaction Award for five consecutive years, and debuted as #288 in *Entrepreneur* magazine's ranking of top 500 franchise systems. Mr. Bongiovanni serves on several local Arizona boards of directors and on the national advisory board of the National Readmissions Prevention Collaborative.

Kerjun Chang, PharmD, received his bachelor of science degree in biochemistry and his doctor of pharmacy degree from the University of Southern California. He has worked with Sheetal Amin at Healthy Living Pharmacy in Yorba Linda, California, to provide clinical services to patients through the implementation of a medication therapy management program in the community setting. He is currently a pharmacist at Palo Verde Hospital in Blythe, California, and is involved in the development and implementation of clinical pharmacy initiatives, including antibiotic stewardship and monitoring.

Kelly Fischer, BSN, CHPN, CHPCA, is chief operating officer at JourneyCare (formerly Hospice and Palliative Care of Northeastern

Illinois) in Barrington, Illinois. In this role, she manages a comprehensive array of programs and services for the agency with a focus on fiscal stewardship and providing excellent clinical care. Previously, she served as a consultant for hospice programs, nursing homes, and long-term care facilities, evaluating and revamping clinical practices and programs while assessing strengths and weaknesses and transforming operations. She earned her bachelor's degree in nursing from Grand Canyon University in Arizona and a diploma in nursing from Flushing Hospital and Medical Center School of Nursing in Queens, New York. She is an active member of the Hospice and Palliative Care National Association and the American Academy of Hospice and Palliative Medicine. She was honored in 2011 with the End-of-Life Nursing Education Consortium's Award of Excellence for Pediatric Palliative Care.

Nicholas Jauregui, MD, is medical director for Supportive Care Medical Group and serves as palliative care medical director for Huntington Hospital in Pasadena, California. Board certified in hospice and palliative medicine, Dr. Jauregui also serves as vice chairman of the ethics committee and chairman of the family medicine section at Huntington Hospital. He earned his bachelor of arts in biology from the University of California, San Diego; went on to earn his medical degree from that institution's School of Medicine; and served his residency at Ventura County Medical Center in Ventura, California.

James S. Kennedy, MD, is a board-certified internal medicine physician trained at the University of Tennessee and credentialed as a certified coding specialist and clinical documentation improvement practitioner by the American Health Information Management Association. As president of CDIMD Physician Champions based near Nashville, Tennessee, Dr. Kennedy and his team support partnerships between physicians and ICD-9-CM / ICD-10 coding professionals that strive toward complete, precise code assignment integral to severity and risk adjustment;

the development of electronic health record infrastructure–promoting ICD-10 documentation and coding compliance; and the defense of provider ICD-9-CM / ICD-10 code assignment with recovery auditors.

Jay Licuanan, MD, owns and operates an internal medicine practice in Lakewood, California, and is vice president and medical director of PA House Calls Medical Group, which helps homebound patients receive quality care medicine at home and helps neighboring hospitals decrease their readmission rates. Dr. Licuanan completed his undergraduate training at California State University, Fullerton; earned his medical degree from the University of Santo Tomas Medical School in the Philippines; and finished his residency training in internal medicine at Overlook Hospital in Summit, New Jersey. He is board certified in internal medicine and is an active member of the American Academy of Internal Medicine, the American Medical Association, and the American Academy of Home Care Physicians.

Sarah Lonowski, MBA, is a second-year medical student at the David Geffen School of Medicine at the University of California, Los Angeles (UCLA). She received her business degree with a customized concentration in healthcare policy and leadership in 2012 from the University of Denver Daniels College of Business. Prior to entering medical school, Sarah worked for a year as the senior project manager for the UCLA Health System Readmission Reduction Initiative led by Dr. Nasim Afsar-manesh.

Adrienne Mihelic, PhD, is a senior biostatistician with Telligen, the Medicare Quality Innovation Network–Quality Improvement Organization for Colorado, Illinois, and Iowa. She provides support to the Advancing Excellence in America's Nursing Homes Campaign under contract with the Centers for Medicare & Medicaid Services. She received her doctoral degree in gerontology and public policy from the University of Southern California and completed a postdoctoral fellowship in the demography and epidemiology of aging at The Johns Hopkins University in Baltimore, Maryland.

Cherilyn G. Murer, JD, CRA, is president and CEO of Murer Consultants Inc., a legal-based healthcare management consulting firm founded in 1985. The firm's client base includes multi-hospital systems, academic medical centers, and large physician group practices. Over the past 30 years, Ms. Murer has coupled her background in law, receiving a JD with honors from Northern Illinois University, with her operational experience as director of rehabilitation medicine at Northwestern Memorial Hospital in Chicago. Ms. Murer is a lecturer and educator focused on helping her clients navigate through the complex regulatory, strategic, and financial issues facing healthcare providers today.

Christine Nesheim, RN, MS, CMAC, is vice president of care management for Lee Memorial Health System, a 1,400-bed multi-hospital system in Fort Myers, Florida. In this role, she is responsible for case management, medical social work, and the system's transfer center and disease management program. The care management department received the American Case Management Association / Joint Commission's Franklin Award of Distinction for exceptional hospital and health system case management in 2005 and the Platinum Award for the Emergency Department Case Management program in 2011. A registered nurse, Ms. Nesheim has more than 25 years of experience in healthcare and has a master's of science degree in human resource development/management and a bachelor of professional studies degree in healthcare administration from Barry University in Miami, Florida.

Debbie Rivet is case management director at Los Alamitos Medical Center in Los Alamitos, California. She started the Preventing Readmissions Collaborative group at Los Alamitos, and her small hospital committee formed to reduce readmissions has now grown to 47 participants, attracting attendees from two counties and numerous agencies. Her 28 years of healthcare experience have made her a leader in the community for case management and readmission efforts, and in 2013 she won the National Readmissions Collaborative Innovator of the Year Award. Originally from Orange, California, she graduated from California State University at Long Beach.

Mariel Sjeime, PharmD, BCACP, is the transition of care pharmacist at Einstein Healthcare Network in Philadelphia, where she focuses on reducing readmission rates in high-risk Medicare patients. She received her doctor of pharmacy degree in 2011 from St. John's University in New York and subsequently completed her PGY-1 pharmacy practice residency at Einstein Medical Center in Philadelphia. During her residency, she developed an interest and strengthened her skills in ambulatory care through work on the outpatient anticoagulation program, immunodeficiency clinic, and Medication REACH program. The Medication REACH program has won awards from Delaware Valley Hospital Council, the Healthcare Improvement Foundation, and the Hospital and Healthsystem Association of Pennsylvania.

Sarah Thomas is a rehabilitation specialist and legislative affairs liaison for Hallmark Rehabilitation in Foothill Ranch, California, and Innovation Fellow for Aging 2.0. Her roles strategically serve to integrate new care delivery models into current and evolving lines of business in the post-acute care sector and along the care continuum. She has been influential in leading culture change for her organization and for other socially responsible organizations in the communities she is involved with. Ms. Thomas has dedicated 15 years to aging services, holding key leadership positions in companies across the country. She combines her occupational therapy degree from Quinnipiac University in Hamden, Connecticut, with her operational, clinical, and entrepreneurial experience to inspire passionate changes to the current systems in the elder care environment.

Alen Voskanian, MD, is regional medical director for VITAS Innovative Hospice Care in California and assistant clinical professor of medicine at the David Geffen School of Medicine at the University of California, Los Angeles (UCLA). He is board certified in hospice/palliative medicine and family medicine and is an HIV specialist certified by the American Academy of HIV Medicine. His primary interest is increasing awareness regarding end-of-life care and addressing the barriers that prevent timely access to hospice and palliative care programs. Dr. Voskanian is a graduate of the University of California, Berkeley and of the University of California, Irvine Medical School. He completed his residency at UCLA and a fellowship in HIV at AIDS Healthcare Foundation. He was selected by the Centers for Medicare & Medicaid (CMS) Center for Medicare & Medicaid Innovation (CMMI) from a pool of more than 900 applicants to be an innovation advisor. His project at CMS/CMMI is based on providing outpatient palliative care to provide better end-of-life care. Dr. Voskanian received the Hasting Center's Cunniff-Dixon Physician Award in 2013 for excellence in end-of-life care.

David G. Wolf, PhD, is CEO of INTERACT T.E.A.M. Strategies, an organization whose mission is to provide the finest training, education, and management consulting services to long-term care facilities seeking to efficiently and effectively implement the INTERACT quality improvement program. He is a certified fellow of the American College of Health Care Administrators (ACHCA) and serves as vice-chair of the mentoring subcommittee and as a board member of ACHCA's Academy of Long-Term Care Leadership and Development. Dr. Wolf graduated with highest honors while earning his master's and doctoral degrees in organizational leadership with a concentration in business strategy. Dr. Wolf has owned and operated nursing homes, assisted-living facilities, rehabilitation centers, home care companies, and nurse staffing agencies.

Barbara J. Zarowitz, PharmD, is the chief clinical officer and vice president of clinical services at Omnicare Inc. and adjunct professor of pharmacy practice at the College of Pharmacy and Health Sciences at Wayne State University and the University of Michigan. She earned her bachelor of science in pharmacy from the University of Toronto; completed her doctor of pharmacy degree and fellowship training at the State University of New York at Buffalo; and spent 21 years with Henry Ford Health System in Detroit, Michigan. At Omnicare, which provides care for 1.4 million elderly nursing home residents and publishes the annual *Geriatric Pharmaceutical Care Guidelines*, a respected source of geriatric pharmacotherapy, Dr. Zarowitz is responsible for creating the organization's clinical mission and developing strategies and tactics to manage drug utilization, including disease management, formulary management, case management, and clinical pharmacy services. She is on faculty at the University of Maryland, Wayne State University, the State University of New York at Buffalo, and the University of Michigan.

Leslie S. Zun, MD, MBA, is system chair of the Department of Emergency Medicine in the Sinai Health System in Chicago and chairman and professor of the Department of Emergency Medicine, with a secondary appointment in the Department of Psychiatry, at the Rosalind Franklin University of Medicine and Science / Chicago Medical School in North Chicago, Illinois. He earned his medical degree from Rush Medical College and his business degree from Northwestern University's Kellogg School of Management. He is board certified by the American Board of Emergency Medicine. His research interests include healthcare administration, violence prevention, and behavioral emergencies. He is a board member of the American Academy of Emergency Medicine and is president-elect of the American Association for Emergency Psychiatry. He is the chief editor of the textbook *Behavioral Emergencies for Emergency Physicians* and has been course director for the past five years of the National Update on Behavioral Emergencies conference.